# Yoga for Real Life

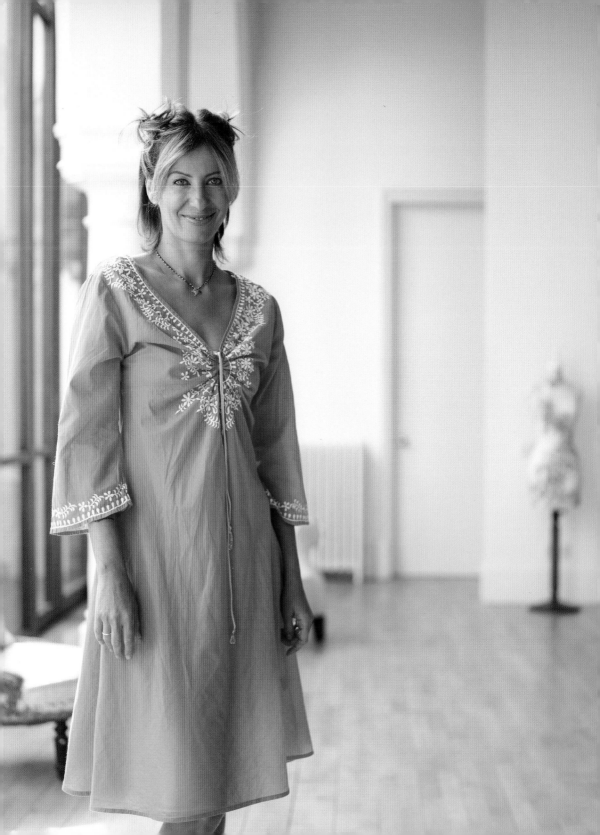

# Yoga for Real Life

## Maya Fiennes

with Sheryl Garratt

Atlantic Books

First published in trade paperback in 2010 by Atlantic Books,
an imprint of Grove Atlantic Ltd.

This paperback edition published in 2012 by Atlantic Books,
an imprint of Atlantic Books Ltd.

10 9 8 7 6

A CIP catalogue record for this book is available from the British Library.

ISBN 978 0 85789 577 6

Designed and typeset by Ghost Design
Photography by David Loftus

Atlantic Books
An imprint of Atlantic Books Ltd
Ormond House
26–27 Boswell Street
London WC1N 3JZ

www.atlantic-books.co.uk

Publisher's note:
Before following any advice or practice suggested in this book, it is recommended that
you consult a doctor as to suitability, especially if you suffer from any health problems or
special conditions. The publishers, the author and the photographer cannot accept
responsibility for any injuries or damage incurred as a result of following the exercises in
this book, or of using any of the therapeutic methods described or mentioned here.

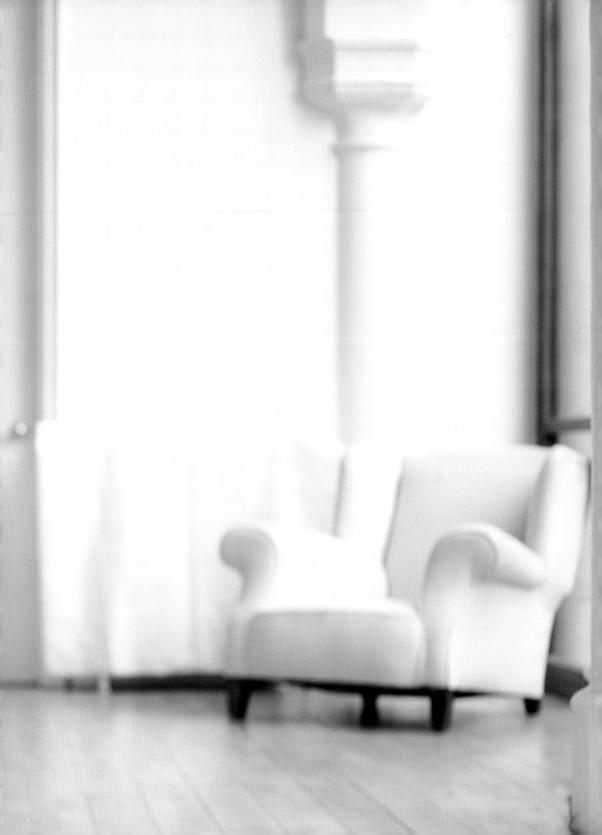

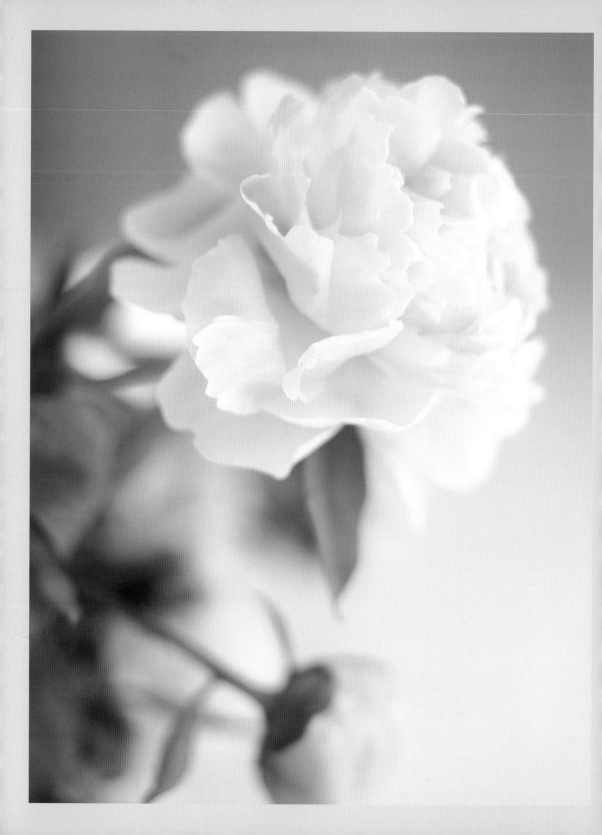

# Contents

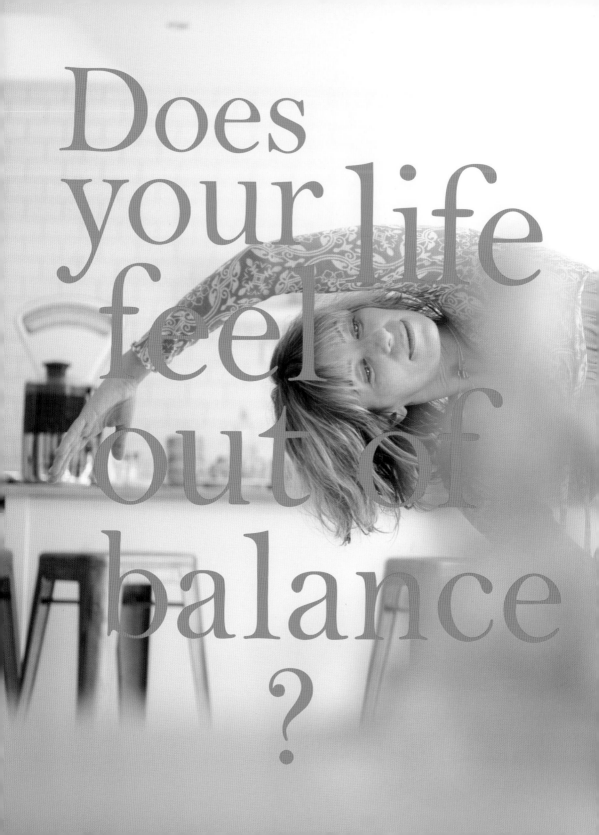

Does your life feel out of balance ?

Would you like to be more relaxed, more able to cope calmly with the stresses of everyday living?

Do you long for more time in your day, to do things without rushing?

Or for a better, deeper relationship with your partner, your family, your friends?

Would you like to look and feel younger, more vibrant and alive?

I believe that Kundalini yoga can do all of this for you and more.

It is something you can introduce easily into a busy life, and it will give you more energy, more creativity, more fun and real peace. What's more, you'll start to feel its benefits almost immediately.

It has changed my life immeasurably for the better, and I know it can change yours.

For me, it is the secret of true joy.

*Maya*

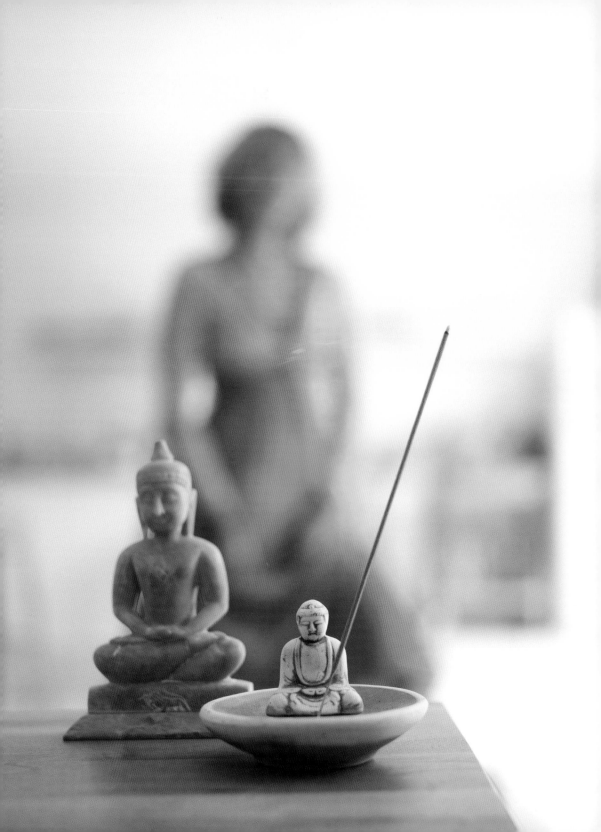

# Introduction

# What is Kundalini yoga?

**THERE ARE MANY TYPES OF YOGA,** and they all have the same goal: to establish unity between breath and movement; body and spirit; between you as an individual and the Universe. That's what the word 'yoga' means: union. Kundalini yoga has its own way of getting you there. It's an ancient technology designed to waken the Kundalini energy we are all born with. It's our essence, our life force, and it lies dormant in the base chakra, at the fourth vertebra of the spine. We need to awaken it if we want to reach our full potential, to become fully conscious and present.

Practising Kundalini can produce powerful and dramatic results very quickly. It lifts your energy levels to new peaks, aligning your whole being until you become more awake, aware and vibrantly healthy. A Kundalini session leaves you feeling fighting fit, ready and able to tackle everyday challenges with new zest. Even if you just do one of the exercises in this book for three minutes, you'll feel some benefit. Do that every day, and you'll quickly start to notice real changes.

A Kundalini session leaves you feeling fighting fit, ready and able to tackle everyday challenges with new zest.

A total workout for the body, mind *and* spirit, Kundalini works by freeing the flow of energy through seven power points in the body known as chakras. The word 'chakra' translates as 'wheel', and perhaps the best way of imagining them is as spinning vortexes at intervals along your spine, each radiating a different energy vibration that's important to your health and happiness. By opening and balancing these centres, we enable ourselves to connect to a larger source of energy, from which we have come, and to which we will return. Kundalini does this with a combination of exercise, chanting and breathing techniques that calm the mind, releasing tension and stress. It builds strength and focus, giving us the spiritual armour we need to survive all that modern living throws at us.

Many of the positions and moves are of themselves quite simple and easy – it is the extended repetition that challenges us. Persevere and you will find new resources of stamina you never imagined. This physical journey, accompanied by chanting and music, is extraordinarily powerful and often quite emotional. Many deep-seated issues and traumas may come to the surface, and it's not unusual to find yourself crying when you first try some of the exercises. It's also very common to feel a real rush as the body's natural painkillers, the endorphins, come surging to help us. I'm used to seeing people cry in my classes, but also to seeing them open up and laugh with pure joy!

Kundalini is about training your mind as well as your body, helping not only the spine to become more flexible but also your attitude to life, balancing the endocrine system that controls our hormone production, and helping us cope with the stresses and challenges of each day more calmly so that we no longer put so much strain on that system.

The word 'Kundalini' – pronounced like the Italian pasta 'linguini' – translates as 'coiled', and the image that is often used to describe the energy lying dormant at the base of our spine is that of a coiled, sleeping serpent. If this sounds intimidating, don't worry. You don't have to go and live in a cave or dedicate your life to it: it can be slotted easily into a working day. You don't need to understand it all to get the full benefit. You don't have to believe it all. Just try it for yourself, and see how you feel. Think of it as a kind of user's manual, a way of troubleshooting problems or simply tuning your body, mind and soul to peak performance.

# A total workout for the body, mind and spirit.

For centuries, the ancient science and technology of Kundalini was a closely guarded secret in India, passed on from master to student over years of study. But in 1969, a devout Sikh called Yogi Bhajan decided to break that secrecy, feeling that it was a much-needed tool for coping with the increasing pressures of life. He went to California with the intention of training teachers to spread Kundalini across the West, and many of his first students were former hippie flower children who found that it gave them the same high, the same feeling of confidence and connectedness that they had been getting from drugs.

We're all looking for more power and energy in our lives, whether we are getting it from food, caffeinated drinks, or taking drugs to enhance our senses momentarily. Kundalini yoga gives me a pure form of energy that seems to radiate from the core connecting my heart, mind and physical being. In this book, I'm hoping to give you the same.

# What do I need to start?

KUNDALINI DOESN'T USE A LOT OF PROPS or expensive equipment. You'll enjoy it most if you're wearing loose, comfortable clothes. You need floor space, and maybe a yoga mat, blanket or rug if the floor is hard. Music is nice: something fast and rhythmic for the more aggressive, active sequences; something relaxing, like a chill-out CD, for the rest. Most of all, you need to bring it your full attention, the commitment to give yourself this time and focus in on yourself, even if only for a few minutes.

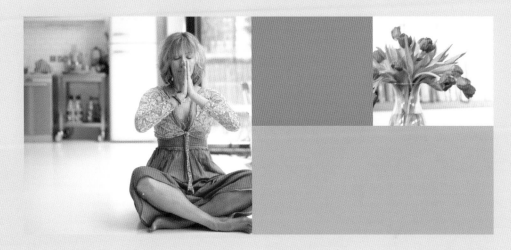

# How to use this book

SOME OF THE THINGS I'M GOING TO ASK YOU TO DO in these pages may seem strange at first. Leave your inhibitions behind, and just see if it works for you. And have fun, smile while you're doing it! I see yoga very much as a celebration of joy and happiness. It shouldn't feel like a chore, or yet another item on your endless to-do list. It's there to help you, to relax you, to build the physical and mental strength you need to live your life to its fullest: it's something we can do, lovingly, for ourselves.

Each of the seven chapters in the book corresponds roughly to one of the chakras, and each chapter offers a selection of postures, meditations, mantra and breathing exercises. I have also created a series of juices and smoothies, designed to enhance the seven energy points. Try them and inspire yourself!

See the exercises in each chapter as a set of tools. You might like to work with just one specific position, meditation or mantra and try doing it for at least three minutes every day for a month or two – you'll notice the changes! In Kundalini we often suggest forty consecutive days as a good time span to commit to. It's a highly symbolic number in many religions, and our bodies renew every cell in the bloodstream every forty days. It is also a long enough time span to make your practice a new habit, and to really feel the benefits of the movement you have chosen.

If you want to build a longer kriya (set of exercises), start with the warm-ups here, or the Five Tibetans described on pages 148–152, then either concentrate on one chakra, or take three or four exercises from different chapters. Do whatever you fancy – the important thing is just to do it! Always end with a meditation or by relaxing in the Corpse Pose described on page 19.

The more often you are able to repeat a movement, and the longer you are able to repeat a mantra or sit in meditation, the more benefit you will receive. Some of you

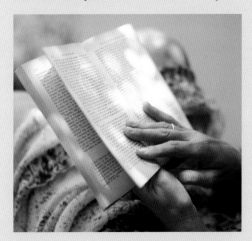

Yogi Bhajan was fond of saying that even if you just lean slightly in the right direction, you'll get some benefit!

will be used to working out and will easily be able to do the full number of repetitions I suggest. In that case, you can do double! Some of you may find it hard doing the more challenging poses even a couple of times at first. There's no hurry: progress at your own pace. Yoga is not about competition, and it's certainly not about screwing up our faces with strain and hurting ourselves. You know your body best, so be gentle and go slowly at the beginning. Follow the instructions and do as much as you can. Remember that breathing,

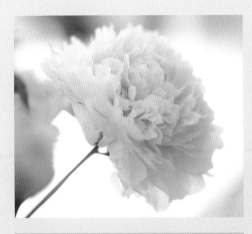

relaxing and staying focused are far more important than pushing your body somewhere it's not yet ready to go.

You may not be able to do the full position at first. That's fine. You'll still get rewards from doing it. Yogi Bhajan was fond of saying that even if you just lean slightly in the right direction, you'll get some benefit! If the instructions tell you to touch your toes and you can barely get your hands to your knees, don't worry. Maybe next time your fingers will reach a little further down. And if you persevere, in a week, a month, or a year you may be bending there easily, but you'll reap the benefits whatever. Just trust the process, enjoy it and believe that you will progress more every day.

There are very few people who won't be able to practise Kundalini yoga. In my classes I've met a woman who was so large she couldn't sit cross-legged comfortably at first, a seventy-two-year-old man from a poor Texan farming family who'd never heard of meditation, a woman with multiple sclerosis who would fall over getting out of bed. All of them found peace, better health and a better quality of life by persevering with Kundalini. However, if you have health problems or have not done any exercise for some time, you may want to see your doctor before you begin this new challenge.

In some exercises, I'll encourage you to push yourself, to put up with tiredness or aching arms for a few seconds more to get the full benefit of a pose. But if you feel any sharp pain or discomfort, please stop. Don't push too hard. Keep reminding yourself that yoga should be fun and enjoyable. It's not supposed to hurt!

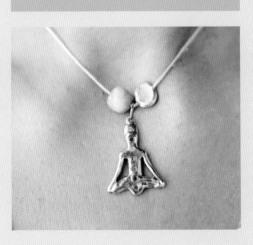

# Before you start

**AS YOU WORK THROUGH THE EXERCISES,** meditations and mantras in this book, you will find that four basic yoga positions crop up repeatedly: Easy Pose, Gyan Mudra, Root Lock and Corpse Pose. As well as being important elements of good Kundalini yoga practice, they can easily be incorporated into everyday activities – and you will find that they even become second nature. Take some time now to familiarize yourself with them – it will pay off in abundance!

## Easy Pose
Sit on the floor or on a mat with your legs crossed comfortably and your back straight, with your shoulders relaxed.

## Gyan Mudra

This is a hand position where you touch your index fingers with your thumbs.

## Root Lock

Suck your navel in, squeezing and pulling up the muscles around your stomach, anus and sex organs to uncoil the Kundalini energy at the base of the spine.

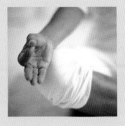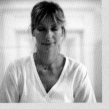

## Corpse Pose

Lie on your back on the floor or on a mat, your hands out to the side with palms facing upwards. Relax your legs, keeping them slightly apart, and let them fall comfortably outwards. If you have lower back problems, you might want to put a pillow or folded blanket under your knees. Tilt your chin slightly down towards your collarbone to lengthen your neck. Now breathe deeply, sink into the floor, and concentrate on releasing and relaxing every part of your body, from your feet to your tongue, eyes and forehead. Then empty your mind by simply concentrating on your breath, observing as it goes in and out. Be open to receiving whatever thoughts and feelings float through you. Relax for as long as you need to. If it helps, you can play soothing, relaxing music.

Afterwards come out of the pose slowly, gently starting to move your hands and toes in a circular motion, first in one direction, then the other. Bend your knees towards your chest and roll over on to your side before opening your eyes and pushing yourself up to a sitting position when you're ready.

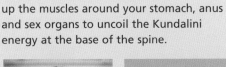

# KUNDALINI YOGA WARM-UP

## A SIMPLE BUT EFFECTIVE DAILY EXERCISE SET

**LET'S LOOK AT A SET OF EXERCISES AND STRETCHES** that can be slipped into your day with minimum fuss. Nothing here is outside the capabilities of even the most sedentary and inexperienced. Kundalini is not about contortion and muscle strain; it's about simple, repetitive moves that gently build stamina, though none of these postures should be considered a mere gymnastic exercise. They are less about the perfectly toned, high-maintenance muscular body, and more about the energized and awakened mind.

You might want to try doing these exercises when you get up in the morning, to loosen your spine and wake up your energy for the day ahead. They will increase the circulation of the spinal fluid, release toxins, and stimulate the twenty-four vertebrae in your spine, increasing their flexibility.

In Kundalini, we almost always inhale and exhale through the nose, keeping the mouth and eyes closed. This encourages a meditative state of mind from which you will achieve a deeper experience of your inner world. Maintain focus on your third eye – the point between your eyebrows – throughout. And don't forget to smile!

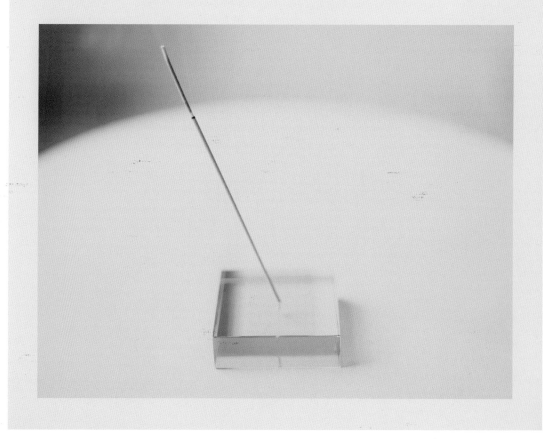

## Spinal Flex

This works on the lower part of the spine, where the Kundalini energy is situated. Sit on the floor or on a mat in Easy Pose (see page 18). Hold your ankles with both hands, and inhale deeply as you flex your spine forward. Lift your chest up, keeping your shoulders relaxed and open. Then, as you exhale, arch your spine backwards. Keep your head parallel to the ground so that it doesn't flop about.

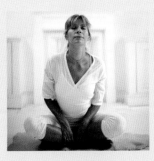

Repeat, synchronizing your breath with the movements to create a rhythm, almost as if you're riding a camel. The deeper you breathe, the more you detoxify. This is your chance to rejuvenate your lungs.

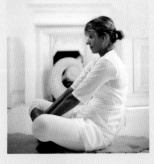

After two or three minutes, come back to the centre in Easy Pose, and inhale. Hold your breath and apply a Root Lock (see page 19). Keep squeezing the muscles, relaxing your shoulders and face, chin slightly in. Hold for about thirty seconds, then release. This pushes the energy up your spine.

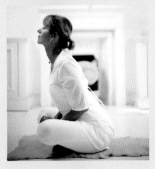

Rest your hands on your knees in Gyan Mudra (see page 19), or put them in a circle in front of you, palms resting on each other, thumbs touching, at your navel point. Take a moment to consolidate, concentrate and focus your energy before starting the next movement.

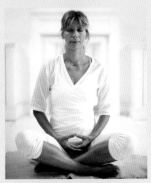

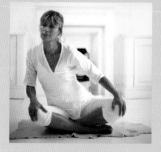

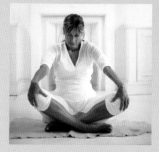

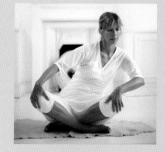

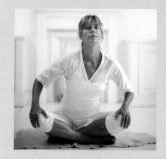

## Sufi Grind

Still sitting in Easy Pose (see page 18), grasp your knees firmly and begin to move your spine in a circular, clockwise movement. Imagine you are drawing a circle around yourself with your chin. Inhale as you bend forward, and exhale as you go backwards. Keep your eyes closed and continue to look between your eyebrows, into your third eye.

After two or three minutes, come back to the centre and start to move in an anti-clockwise direction for the same amount of time. This movement is very soothing – you'll feel yourself becoming one with everything around you that makes that orbital movement, from the planets to the cells in your body.

After two or three minutes, come back to the centre and apply a Root Lock (see page 19). Imagine the Kundalini energy pushing up, clearing all the blockages on the way, until it reaches the crown chakra at the top of your head and establishes a union with the Universe.

After about thirty to sixty seconds, release and relax completely. Put your hands in Gyan Mudra (see page 19), and take a moment to adjust to any changes. If at any point you need to stretch your legs for a minute, please do.

## Spinal Twist

This position stimulates the lower and mid-spine, and massages your internal organs. Remain cross-legged in Easy Pose (see page 18). Hold your shoulders with your fingers in front, thumbs at the back. Inhale and twist to the left, exhale and twist to the right. Keep your elbows high, your arms parallel to the ground. Repeat, doing the movement in your own time and slowly building speed as you feel more comfortable with the twist, co-ordinating it with your breath. As we are bringing in a lot of oxygen, making chemical changes in the blood and releasing endorphins, you will get a real high, and you may also feel a little light-headed at first. If this happens, simply slow down, or rest. It will only happen the first few times, while you get used to it.

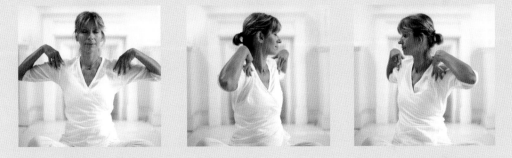

After two or three minutes, put your hands into Gyan Mudra (see page 19) and continue twisting. With every twist raise your arms slightly higher. You'll now feel different muscle groups working. When you reach the top, you will feel a pulling under your armpits, stimulating and cleansing the lymph glands. Keep breathing evenly.

After one minute, inhale and bring your hands into a prayer pose above your head. Stretch, hold – and relax your arms down, hands still in prayer pose, for a minute. In this minute we breathe, we pulse and we regenerate. Our hearts beat, our minds create and our souls digest. Just one minute such as this, well used, is worth a lifetime.

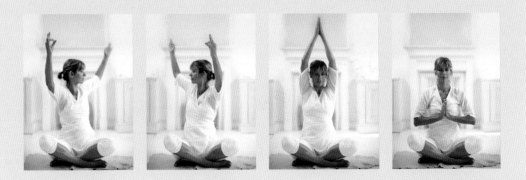

## Neck Rolls

Still sitting in Easy Pose (see page 18), begin rolling your neck very gently in a clockwise, circular motion. Inhale when your head is back, and exhale when it is forward. Take it slowly. This exercise stimulates the thyroid, parathyroid, pituitary and pineal glands, responsible for releasing hormones and regulating a variety of bodily functions, and gives harmony to the entire body. After a couple of minutes, come back to the centre and do the same exercise in the opposite direction.

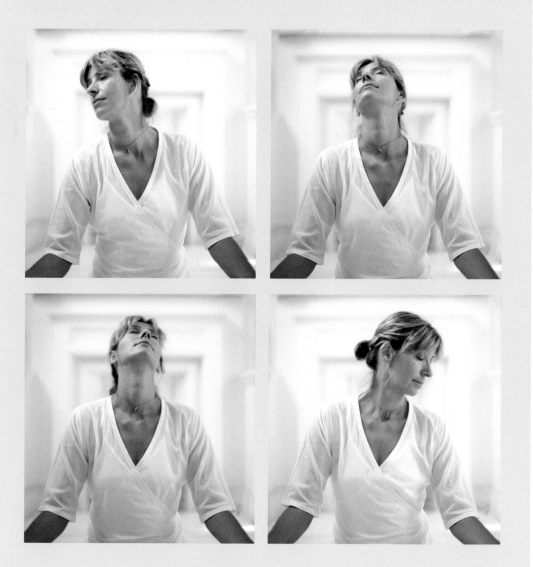

## Life Nerve Stretch

Sit on the floor with your legs stretched wide apart. With your arms above your head, inhale, hold, and then exhale. Stretch down and, if you can, grab the toes of your left foot. If not, just go as far down your leg as you can. Inhale, straighten up, then exhale and stretch down over your right leg. Continue for one to three minutes.

Now bring your hands down to the ground and immediately bring your legs together. Stretch your arms up above your head as you inhale, and come forward to grab your toes – or as far down your leg as you can reach – as you exhale. Breathe normally as you hold the pose. This exercise is deeply relaxing, as it allows the glandular secretions to circulate through the body. Stay in this position for about two minutes, or as long as is comfortable. Then inhale, come up and release your hands.

Go into Easy Pose (see page 18), close your eyes, put your hands in Gyan Mudra (see page 19) and relax for a couple of minutes before continuing with your session.

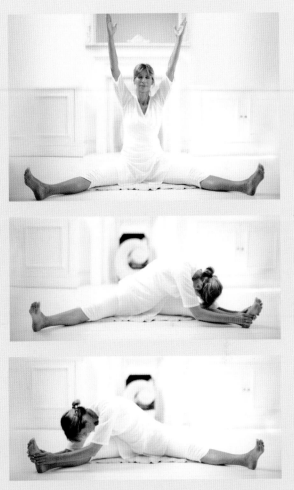

## Corpse Pose

If this is all you want to do for now, finish by relaxing for a few minutes in Corpse Pose (see page 19). This is one of the most important positions in yoga, also known as savasana (pronounced shah-vahs-ana). Some teachers say it is one of the most challenging, because it's so hard for us to relax completely without falling asleep! Yoga classes will nearly always end with this pose: it is when the body processes the information it has received, rests and absorbs the changes and the healing.

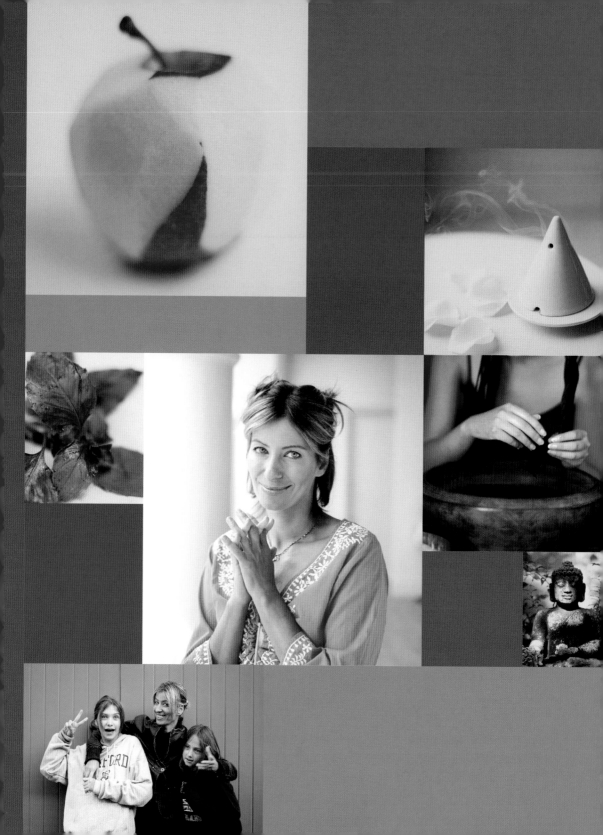

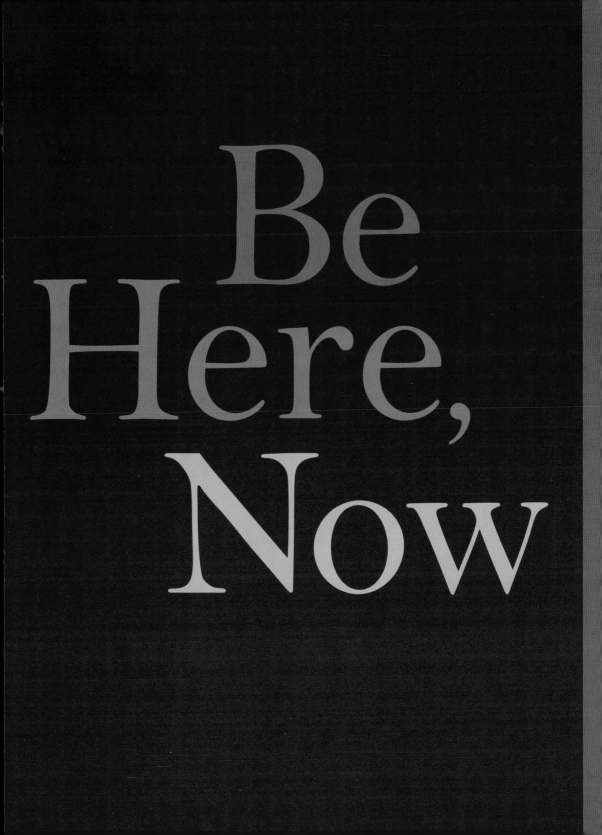

Be
Here,
Now

# ROOT CHAKRA

THIS FIRST CHAKRA IS SITUATED at the base of the spine, where the Kundalini energy lies dormant. It is connected to the organs of elimination and is the foundation of everything in our lives. As every builder knows, you have to dig deep through the accumulated muck and dirt to build strong foundations! All our fears are stored here, so if you don't clear it, you'll live a fearful life. All our habits and addictions come from this area too, and you need to do quite aggressive and physical positions to clear it, working on the legs because you need to be grounded.

Once you've cleared the energy points of blockages, you'll start to grow in confidence. You'll begin to accept and love yourself exactly the way you are. And then you'll accept that everything is as it is – and that it is perfect, at that moment. So first you accept yourself, and then you accept the way life is, and you don't fight it: instead you go with it, flow with it. And very often, later on, you'll find, 'Wow! I was so worried about that, and now I realize I shouldn't have been, because look where it brought me.' As you start clearing the energy, clearing the chakras, you will find that this flow comes ever more easily.

The first three chakras are closely interconnected, and together are known as the lower triangle. They all focus on elimination, on getting rid of dead energy and waste matter, and their elements of earth, water and fire work closely together.

| GOVERNS: | SHADOW EMOTIONS: | COLOUR: | SYMBOL: | ELEMENT: |
|---|---|---|---|---|
| Acceptance, confidence and security | Resentment, rigidity | Red | A lotus with four petals | Earth |

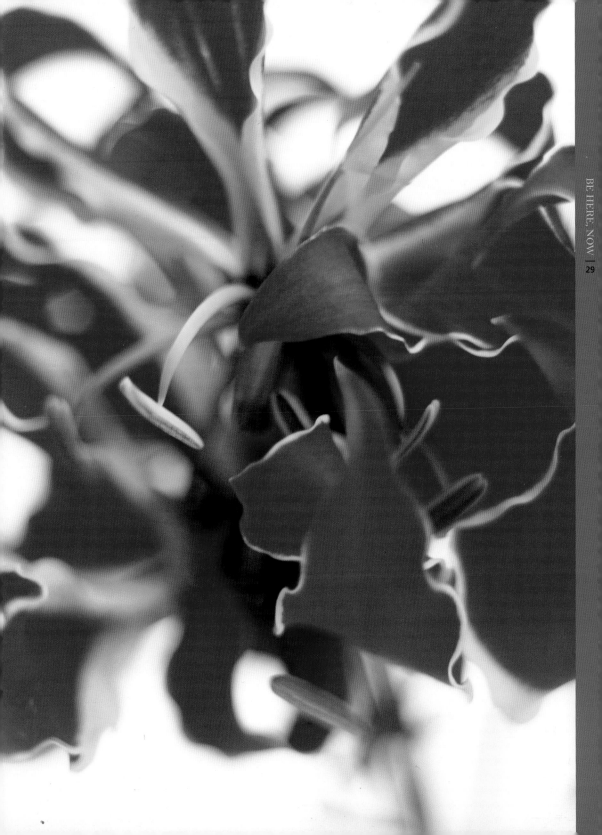

# Living in the moment

'Every morning, when we wake up, we have twenty-four brand new hours to live. What a precious gift!' THICH NÂHT HANH (b.1926)

IF THERE IS A SINGLE SKILL you should learn in order to guarantee a full, happy, healthy, meaningful life, it is this. Be here, now. Be present and aware. Live in the moment. That's easy to say, of course, and far harder to do in our everyday lives. We all have memories of being on holiday, watching the sun set over the sea or the mountains, and the sense of awe and wonder we get as the sky lights up in shades of red, pink and gold, that feeling of peace and connectedness. Yet the sun sets every day when we're at home, too, and we barely notice.

We lead increasingly busy lives, juggling work, family, chores and all the other things on our seemingly endless to-do list, while being bombarded with an ever-growing amount of information and distractions. We have hundreds of TV channels, too many magazines for even the biggest newsagent's to display, while shops and supermarkets have such a wide selection of goods that sometimes the choice can be overwhelming. And with the internet, the amount of information, entertainment and goods available grows by the day. Nor does it stop when we look away from the screen. Those phone calls, texts and emails keep coming now, even when we're on the move. In many ways, these technologies have made our lives better. But most of us have a nagging feeling that something is missing. And that something is often you.

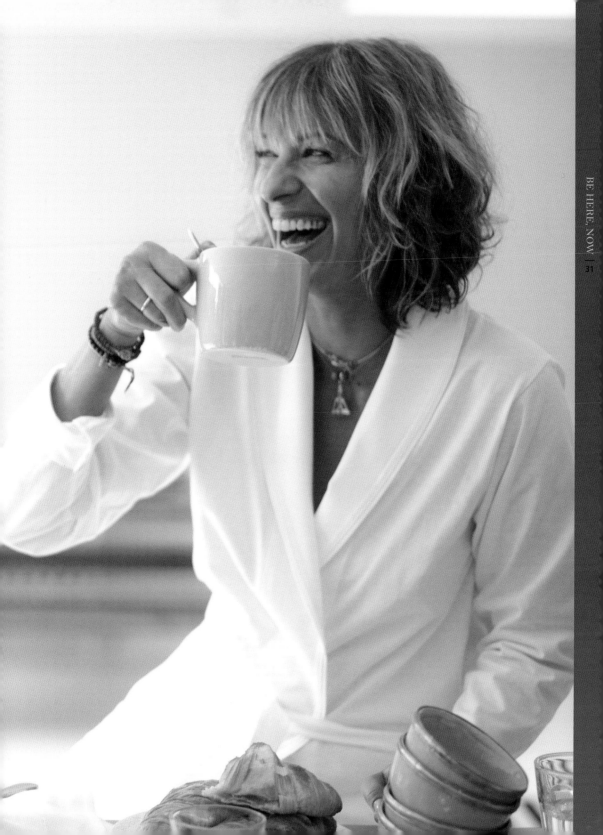

We're so busy rushing ahead to the next thing, trying to multitask and listening to the endless stream of chatter in our minds, that we miss the magic around us here and now. A mum rushing to pick up her kids from school, still talking to someone in the office on her mobile while waving hello to other parents and deciding what she's going to cook for dinner, can easily miss seeing the way her child's face lights up as he runs out of class towards her. Commuters can be so preoccupied with getting to work that they don't notice the first daffodils opening in the park beside the station, let alone take a second to really appreciate their beauty, or to smile because spring is nearly here. Others are so busy trying to record that concert, party or holiday on video to watch later that they forget to actually enjoy it while it's happening.

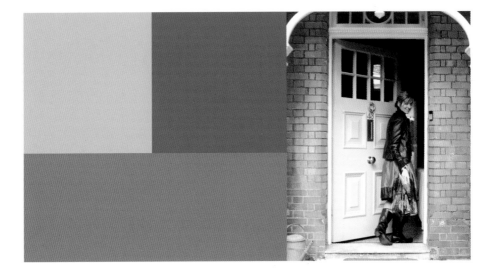

We've all seen these people. We've all *been* these people.

So how do we change? We do the easiest, most natural thing in the world. We just breathe.

Stop. Take a deep, cleansing breath. In fact, treat yourself, take a few more. Air is free, yet we're often shockingly mean with how much we allow ourselves to have. Now take a moment to look around you – use all your senses, in fact. Notice where you are, what is happening, how you are feeling. And smile!

Bringing yourself back into the present is that simple. What's difficult is remembering to do it when the phone is ringing, or you're late for work, or you're in the express queue in the supermarket and you've just noticed that the person before you has way, way more than ten items in their basket.

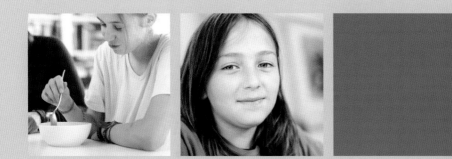

We forget ourselves all the time because we're too wrapped up in the stories we are busy running through our heads. We find it hard to be in the present because we're still trapped in the past, re-running old grievances, love affairs, things we wish we'd said or done or regret saying or doing. Either that or we're running ahead of ourselves into the future, planning what we're going to here, now, in this moment. In religious communities, bells are often sounded at certain times of day to remind people to pray or meditate, to silence their mental chatter. Unless you're planning to become a monk or nun any time soon, you might want to think of more everyday things that will remind you to come back to that moment. When you're driving, for instance, you could get into

## Stop. Take a deep, cleansing breath. In fact, treat yourself, take a few more.

do tonight, this weekend, this summer, when we win the lottery. We can't change the past. We can't control the future. We can't control the present either, but we do get to choose how we *react* to what is going on around us, how we feel about it – and that often affects what happens next.

So keep asking yourself these questions. Where am I, right now? *Here*. Who am I, at this moment? *Myself*. What's the time? *Now*. It all leads to that: the habit of taking a few deep breaths every time you stop at a red light. You won't take any longer to get where you're going, but you might arrive a lot less stressed! Waiting for a bus, queuing in a shop, all those random, repetitive tasks you do at work – photocopying, waiting for a computer to reboot, using a specific tool or piece of equipment – can be used as opportunities, reminders to quieten all that mental chatter and just open yourself up to the here and now.

Kundalini, and the root chakra exercises in this chapter, will help ground you in the present. One of my students, Jacqui, still remembers her first session vividly. 'Afterwards I felt like skipping down the road. I just felt filled with energy, and so happy. I've never taken drugs, but I'm sure that must be how it feels to be high! Everything just seemed more real somehow, more vibrant, like moving from black and white into colour. Food tasted better, music sounded amazing, I felt so alive to everything around me.'

Once you start to bring yourself back into the present more often, you begin to treasure those mundane moments that make an ordinary day feel extraordinary. One of the biggest luxuries you can give yourself in the middle of a hectic day is the luxury of time. It doesn't have to be much. A few minutes to sit on the grass and reconnect with nature, a few seconds to smile and say hello to those people you see every day but often fail to notice: a near neighbour, a shop assistant, that woman who works two floors below your office whom you often see in the lift.

Next time you're walking somewhere, try switching off your mobile, taking off your headphones, and just for once stop running through your endless mental to-do list. Instead just acknowledge the trees as you pass them, admire a pretty window-box or a well-kept garden, notice that cat warming itself in a ray of winter sun. Listen to the birds singing or the sound of laughter drifting from an open window. Enjoy the rhythm of your feet against the ground, of your own breathing. And see how much better you feel when you get to your destination!

You need a little confidence to become comfortable with this. To know that the world isn't going to stop turning if you don't dash to answer the phone immediately, if you stop to smell the flowers or the coffee, or if you look someone in the eyes and really *listen* to what they're saying instead of tidying your desk, checking your texts or putting the toys away at the same time. Just be present, for that moment, enjoy it, and let it go... And then, there's another moment.

Give yourself time to breathe. Tell yourself, 'I owe it to myself. I can do this for myself.' Then your tantra, your way of living, becomes different: you're calmer, and you create a different environment around yourself. You no longer create chaos.

# Learning to receive

'If a man insisted always on being serious, and never allowed himself a bit of fun and relaxation, he would go mad or become unstable without knowing it.'
HERODOTUS (c.484 – c.425 BC)

A WHILE AGO, I MET A COACH WHO WORKS WITH LONG-DISTANCE RUNNERS. He told me that between an athlete's morning run and his evening workout, the most important thing he can do to help his training is rest completely – and that means staying off his feet and doing nothing. Many of his athletes are of African descent, but they grew up in Europe and have problems with this. To them, 'doing nothing' means going to the shops, meeting friends, doing chores. To their coach, it means sitting with your feet up and not moving at all. He encouraged one of his elite runners to share a house with some runners from the Kenyan national team for a while so that he could learn how the best distance runners in the world live and train – and especially how they switch off after a run, allowing the body to rest and absorb what it has learned. 'Africans still understand stillness,' explained the coach. 'They've mastered the art of doing nothing. It's something we've lost in the West.'

We are all good at adding more work to our day, but not so good about allowing ourselves time to rest. We feel guilty, selfish and lazy if we take time off from our constant busyness, as if we're wasting precious time. Yet we're human beings, not human doings, and unless we allow ourselves to recuperate, to just be, we're no good to anyone.

In yoga we balance the yang, the masculine energy of doing, of action, with the yin, the female energy of stillness, of receiving. When doing a set of Kundalini exercises, it's important to take a few seconds between poses to just rest with your palms open or with your index finger and thumb touching in Gyan Mudra (see page 19) – the hand position you often see on Buddha statues. The index fingers represent the planet Jupiter, for knowledge, the thumbs represent planet Earth. Touching them together allows us to receive knowledge and connect with our inner wisdom.

At the end of a yoga class, we always rest for a while in Corpse Pose (see page 19. Sometimes people rush off, feeling they've done the exercise and can skip this bit, but the relaxation is the most important part. Lie in Corpse Pose for at least five minutes for every thirty minutes you've spent on the poses. After changing your energies, clearing the chakras, you have to allow a few minutes so that everything settles and the energy is distributed properly around the body. It's so important, otherwise we just work, work, work, achieve and achieve, and then we're off to the next thing, forgetting to enjoy what we've done.

Very often, in our Western lifestyle, we don't allow time for silence, emptiness and quietness in our lives, but that's when we receive energy, inspiration – when we plug ourselves in to the source. And we really have to be more mindful of that. Even if it's just for a few minutes, stop, be silent, do nothing. And see how much more you achieve in your day afterwards.

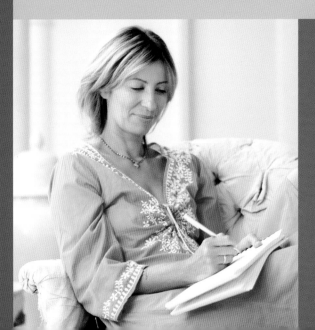

Very often, in our Western lifestyle, we don't allow time for silence, emptiness and quietness.

# Counting your blessings

'Gratitude is not only the greatest of virtues,
but the parent of all others.'
CICERO (106–43 BC)

WHEN I WAKE UP in the morning, before I even get out of bed, I take a couple of minutes just to be grateful, to say thank you for being who I am, for being alive. To me, there's no better way to start the day. It's very simple. You don't have to go into huge detail. You don't even have to mean it, at first. Force yourself. Just say it. After a few days, you'll find you really start appreciating. And then you'll start saying it for real.

*think*. Be grateful for your family and friends. For the water you're using to shower or brush your teeth. For the fact that the sun is shining, or the rain is giving the trees and plants a revitalizing drink. Every day, we get a choice. We can fixate on petty resentments about everything that's gone wrong with our day, or we can look instead for everything that's gone right. Celebrate the little things: a baby's laugh, a beautiful sky, a joke, a stranger offering a kind hand.

## Say thank you for being who you are, for being alive. To me, there's no better way to start the day.

If you keep a diary or a journal, try writing down five things you're thankful for, every day. If writing isn't your thing, just list them in your head at a certain point in your day: while you're brushing your teeth, for instance, or in the shower. If you're feeling really low, you might find this difficult. You might feel you have nothing to be grateful for. But there's always something. You are alive. You are breathing. You most likely have all your fingers and toes. You can see, hear, taste, smell, and feel. You can

It's human nature not to be appreciative of what we have. We take so much for granted. There may be times when you feel there is little to be grateful for. Those are exactly the moments that test you. When everything is fine and beautiful, it's easy to be grateful. When things are more challenging, you need to trust, to have faith. Say thank you, and things will change.

# Letting go of fear and doubt

WE CAN BE VERY SCARED OF CHANGE, and the first chakra is all about change, about losing our rigidity and learning to be more flexible. That's why this chakra is also very connected to addiction – because addiction is based on fear, a complete fear of living, of feeling.

Fear is something we all have. It's part of being alive, and of knowing that some day all of us will die. We're never going to lose fear completely, so we need to learn how best to deal with it. We need be able to acknowledge it, accept it, recognize it, admit to it – and then let it go.

In Macedonia, where I grew up, we have a saying: 'Better the devil you know than the angel you don't know.' As I've travelled the world, I've found that most places have a version of it. We're all afraid of the unknown. So we stay in a relationship that doesn't work any more, because we're afraid of being alone. Or we keep doing a job we hate, because we're scared we won't find another one.

We are often afraid of failing, but what is worse, to try and fail, or not to try at all? As the great inventor Thomas Edison said, 'If I find 10,000 ways something won't work, I haven't failed. I am not discouraged, because every wrong attempt discarded is another step forward.' And without Mr Edison, we wouldn't have the light bulb!

'Courage is resistance to fear, mastery of fear – not absence of fear.'
MARK TWAIN (1835–1910)

Yoga is a tool for dealing with anxiety. Are you going to let your fear paralyse you, and mean that you never try anything in life because it's scary? If you feel it's better to do nothing, what kind of living is that? You miss out!

Sarah contacted me soon after trying out my first Kundalini DVD, and she's agreed to share her story here. In her mid-twenties, she went to see a naturopathic doctor about a niggling lower back pain, and he assaulted her. Later, she discovered he wasn't a qualified doctor at all. The attack left her with health problems that she now believes were created mainly by extreme fear and anxiety. She developed increasingly serious stomach complaints, until she was no longer able to digest food unless it was almost liquid. Doctors were unable to do anything to relieve her symptoms, and then, after a couple of years, she began struggling for breath. 'I was fighting for air all the time,' she says. 'It was like when you're in a panic. All the doctors could suggest were anxiety pills, but I didn't want to go on heavy medication. I was so young – this was just the beginning of my life! And they were telling me I wouldn't be able to eat or breathe.'

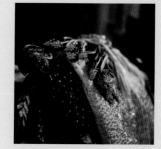

She did her first Kundalini session after yet another anxious, sleepless night, and just after finishing the warm-ups she found herself sobbing uncontrollably. 'It released the tension from my diaphragm, and I took in my first full breath for the first time in months. It gave me faith that I'd be able to breathe again. I slept soundly that night and the next day I was so exhausted I didn't get out of bed – I felt like I'd run a marathon.'

Sarah has continued doing Kundalini exercises daily, and has now trained to be a teacher herself. 'I'm an entirely different person now,' she laughs. 'I still have some health problems, but nowhere near as bad as they were, and I use my yoga as a way of helping my body heal itself. If my stomach isn't digesting, I'll do breathing exercises, and I no longer feel the same fear, anxiety and despair. I'm back now, and life is really good.'

She can find humour in the encounter with the fake doctor, and says that in some ways she is even grateful for it. 'If it hadn't happened, I wouldn't have discovered Kundalini, and I can't imagine my life without it now.'

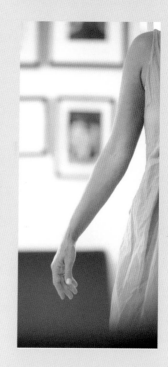

# Meditation for beginners

ANYTHING YOU DO WITH AWARENESS IS MEDITATION. Just quietly concentrating on and observing your own breathing is meditation. Listening to music can be meditation, as can knitting, walking, cleaning. As long as an activity is free from any other distraction to the mind, it is effective meditation. But there are still huge benefits in taking time out every day to sit quietly and clear your mind of all its clutter. There is no better way of learning to live in the present, of realizing that all our fears and worries are just thoughts, and that if we want to, we can let them go. Just five minutes will do at first, although once you start to feel the benefits you may want to do more.

## As long as an activity is free from any other distraction to the mind, it is effective meditation.

The whole point of yoga, of the asanas or positions, is to help us to be more flexible so that we can sit cross-legged for a longer time to meditate. We meditate to find peace, bliss, and happiness – to find that human-ness within. It's all about balance. The yang is masculine, all about action and doing. So we need that feminine part, the yin, which is stillness.

There are many ways to get into meditation, and the simplest is just to sit. Sit, and clear your mind of thoughts. Of course, that's far harder than it sounds, because as soon as you try all the thoughts will come rushing in like crazy! Kundalini yoga has many different ways of helping you focus and enjoy the benefits of meditation, and you'll be practising them as you work through these pages. Thoughts will always creep in, but with practice you will learn to observe them from a distance – like a TV screen flickering in a room across the street – rather than getting involved in whatever story they're telling you. When you meditate, everything stops. Even though you may have your eyes closed, you can see clearly, within. You rejuvenate, re-energize, connect with the flow of life. I often used to notice that same feeling when I played a concert as a professional pianist. When I'm performing, I don't hear. I don't think. It all becomes at peace. Suddenly I'm in a different zone, and everything is quiet. It's an amazing feeling, and anyone can tap into it, any time. We just have to know how.

# TIPS

## WASHING UP MINDFULLY

IT'S EASY TO BE PRESENT WHEN YOU'RE DOING SOMETHING YOU LOVE. But chores are a great way of practising mindfulness. Don't resent it. Don't rush it. Tell yourself you're going to enjoy this. Put on some relaxing music. Enjoy the feeling of the warm water on your hands, the colours in the bubbles. Look at each plate or dish. Be aware of the dish, the water, the movement of your hands. You are cleaning the dishes. You are making them shiny and new again. You are doing this as an act of love for your family, your flatmates, the friends you ate with, yourself. You are acknowledging the people who made the dishes, who grew and made the food you've just eaten. It may seem a little *Stepford Wives* at first, but go with it, just be there in the moment and see how it feels.

'If I am incapable of washing dishes joyfully, if I want to finish them quickly so that I can go and have dessert, I will be equally incapable of enjoying my dessert,' says the Vietnamese monk and teacher Thich Nhât Hanh. 'With my fork in my hand, I will be thinking about what to do next, and the texture and flavour of the dessert, together with the pleasure of eating it, will be lost. I will always be dragged into the future, never able to live in the present moment.'

This works for all chores. If you can be present when you're doing the vacuuming or scrubbing the bath, you will also be more able to appreciate and enjoy it when great moments come along!

## KEEPING YOUR TEMPER

WE ALL HAVE OUR PRESSURE POINTS. One of mine is being in the car, doing the school run. You know how damaging that can be for your psyche! It's raining, the kids are fighting, there's the traffic – drivers can be so aggressive, screaming and shouting at each other. So I like to play mantras in the car. When I give a lift to someone who doesn't know me well, they'll say, 'There's something wrong with your CD. It keeps repeating!'

When you feel yourself losing it, when you're just spinning and spinning, you need to stop, acknowledge it, and decide, 'OK, now I'm going to change this.' Even if you just breathe consciously, it stops, and you don't feel you'll lose your temper any more. It changes. It reverses. Everything that goes down has to go up. And the other way round. You have to just stop and acknowledge it.

Rather than screaming, try closing your right nostril with your right index finger, with your left hand raised with left ring finger and thumb touching, then breathing hard and noisily, inhaling and exhaling for an equal amount of time. By breathing through the left nostril only, you are bringing in calming, female moon energy rather than the invigorating, masculine sun energy that enters on the right-hand side. You may feel a bit ridiculous doing this in the car, but trust me, to other motorists the sight of you red-faced and shouting at the kids is even more absurd. Even if you only do it for a minute, it can change the way you feel.

## The Connector

This drink will cleanse your liver, kidneys and bowels, and will help you reconnect in harmony with Mother Earth.

3 carrots
1 beetroot
1 lemon
1 cucumber
1 red pepper
1 stick of celery
fresh root ginger, to taste
garlic, to taste
small bunch of fresh parsley

Peel the carrots, beetroot, lemon and cucumber. Remove the stalk and seeds from the red pepper. Add ginger and garlic to taste, and put everything through a juicer. Stir, and enjoy with passion!

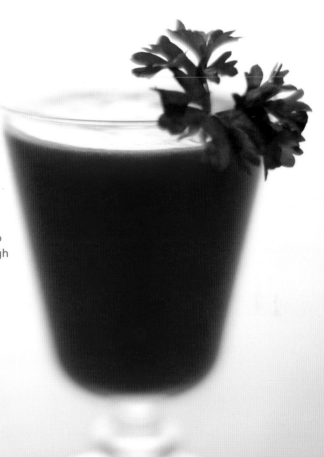

## Moving Crow Pose

This position is very strengthening, both physically and mentally. It stimulates your Kundalini energy and shifts it up your spine. It grounds you to that place of total self-acceptance and letting go. Do not do it, however, if you are pregnant or during the first three days of your period.

Sit in Crow Pose: squatting with feet apart. Extend your arms in front of you and clasp your hands, with the index fingers pointing straight ahead. Inhale through the nose as you rise up into a standing position, keeping your arms parallel to the ground. Exhale through the nose and come back down into a squat. When you inhale, rising up, mentally recite the mantra 'Sat', and when you exhale, mentally recite 'Nam' – meaning 'Truth is my name'. Keep your eyes just a fraction open.

Repeat at least seven times, building up to twenty-six times. As you become stronger and more flexible, you'll be able to do the movement faster, staying in the rhythm of your breath.

If you find this position too difficult, lean your back against a wall to get into the basic squat position, or put two heavy chairs either side of you as supports. Stay there as long as you can – it will become easier and more comfortable the more you practise. In the developing world, where armchairs aren't so easy to find, even elderly people will relax in a squat.

## Frog Pose

This position is connected to facing up to fear of failure. It tunes all the organs of the body, and is excellent for reducing the risk of breast and prostate cancer. It is also good for circulation and for raising the energy from the lower to the higher chakras. Practise it regularly and you'll find yourself more able to let go, to trust and accept. You should also avoid creaky knees as you get older!

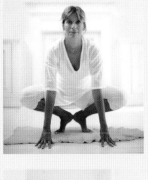

Squat on your toes, heels raised off the ground and touching each other, legs splayed out to the side like a frog. With eyes closed, place your hands on the ground and focus your attention on the third eye, rolling your eyes up to look between your eyebrows. Breathe in and straighten your legs, raising your buttocks, hands remaining on the ground. Your heels should remain off the ground. Breathe out, and return to the squat. Repeat at least seven times, building up to twenty-six times. Again, you can build up speed as you get used to the position.

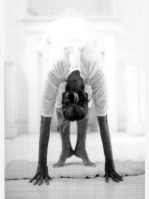

You'll really sweat when you're doing this pose or the Moving Crow Pose (opposite). But afterwards you'll feel that your head is clear and you can let go, you can get on with life.

## Grounding

Lie on your back. Bring your knees to your chest and hug them as you inhale. Sit up, stretch your legs out and grab your toes. Exhale and come back to your original position. Continue for one to two minutes in a steady rhythm.

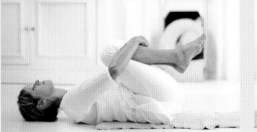
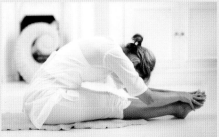

## Fresh start mantra

You may feel embarrassed or uncomfortable chanting out loud, and we deal with that more fully in the next chapter. But do try this if you want to make real changes in your life. It is used to remove blockages in life and dispel old energies that are holding you back.

Mantra is the sound vibration and rhythmical repetition of sacred words of empowerment, which elevate your consciousness. This mantra invokes the Kundalini energy to give you vitality and purify your past karma. It's the mantra of ecstasy, which allows you the experience of going from darkness to light, from ignorance to true understanding. Chanting it out loud stimulates the reflex points in the mouth and then hits the hypothalamus, pineal and pituitary glands to neutralize your mind. It puts you in a meditative state of mind and you experience peace.

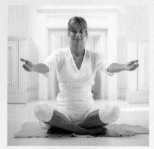

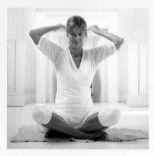

Sit cross-legged in Easy Pose (see page 18). Extend both arms in front of you with the palms facing up, then move both arms together as if you were splashing water over your head, while repeating the mantra, 'Wahe guru, wahe guru, wahe guru, wahe jio' (*wah-hey goo-roo, wah-hey jee-oh* – you can hear it on my website, at www.mayaspace.com). Continue for at least three minutes.

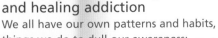

## Releasing fear, breaking habits and healing addiction

We all have our own patterns and habits, things we do to dull our awareness: email, television, shopping. If we are not addicted to smoking, eating or drinking then we are addicted to rejection and fear of failure, all of which lead us to insecure and neurotic behaviour patterns. This meditation corrects this problem. It is excellent for everyone, but particularly effective for rehabilitation efforts in drug dependence, mental illness and phobic conditions. The pressure exerted by the thumbs triggers a rhythmic reflex current into the central brain, which activates the pineal gland. It is the imbalance in this area that makes fear unbreakable.

Sit cross-legged in Easy Pose (see page 18). Make fists with both hands, with extended thumbs. Press your thumbs firmly on your temples. Lock your back molars together, keeping your lips closed. Keeping your teeth pressed together, squeeze your back teeth tightly, then release the pressure. You'll be able to feel the muscle moving under your thumbs. With every squeeze, silently vibrate the sounds 'Sa, ta, na, ma' (*saah taah naah maah* – listen to it at www.mayaspace.com). Do this every day for forty days, and you will be transformed.

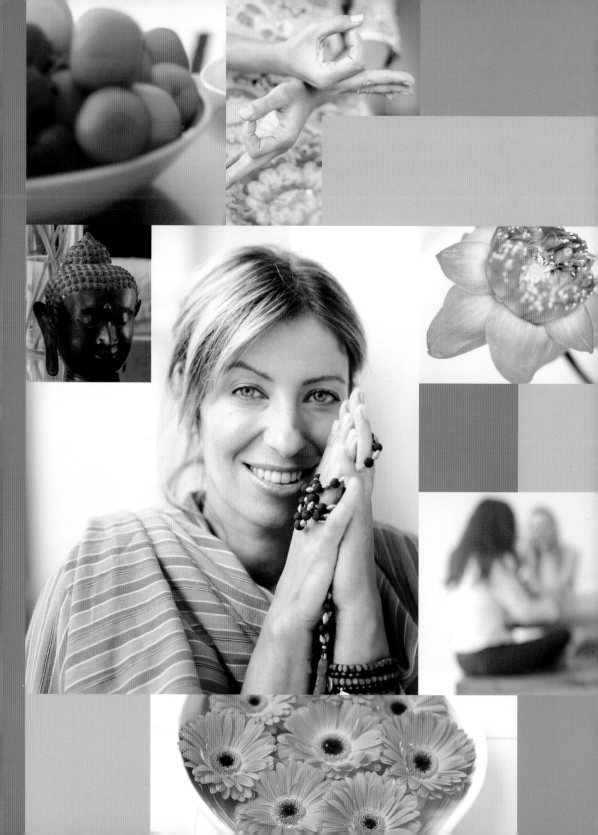

# Detox & De-Stress

# SACRAL CHAKRA

THE SECOND CHAKRA IS LOCATED IN THE SACRUM, the bone that connects your lumbar spine to your tailbones and lower pelvis. It corresponds to the reproductive organs, kidneys and adrenals. Its element is water, and it's all about flow and flexibility towards life. Our children and everything else we create comes from this energy centre.

I meet many passionate but frustrated people who never seem to achieve what they are capable of. They have an immense love of life and its possibilities, yet are continuously disappointed that they cannot manifest them. Others have the opposite problem: they feel tired, impotent and unable to drum up the enthusiasm needed to make a difference in their lives. But once the energies in this chakra are rebalanced, creativity and passion flow with ease in their lives again.

Imbalance in this area could lead to sex addiction or other psychological disorders which give us thrills that seemingly satisfy our fertile imaginations, but ultimately leave us feeling empty and incomplete. Other associated problems include shame about our body or sexuality, impotence, frigidity, infertility, urinary problems and lower back pain.

GOVERNS:
Creativity

SHADOW EMOTIONS:
Sexual problems, shame, guilt and jealousy

COLOUR:
Orange

SYMBOL:
A lotus with six petals

ELEMENT:
Water

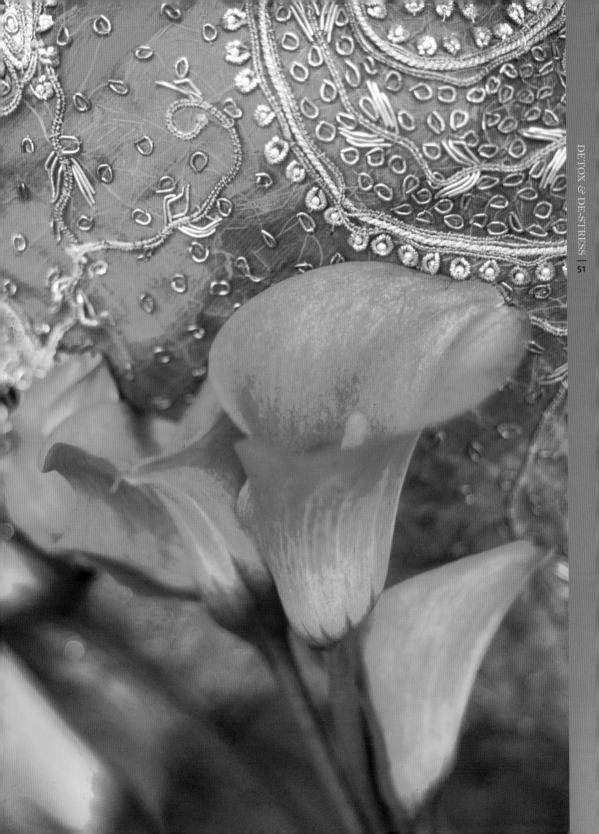

# Stress and how to deal with it

DO YOU OFTEN FEEL COMPLETELY OVERWHELMED? Are you permanently tired, snappy, prone to catch every cold, bug and infection that's going round? Do you worry constantly, or feel there's never enough time in the day to get everything done? If you're also suffering from insomnia, if you're often anxious or moaning and you're having difficulty with the most basic decisions, it's time to see that red flag, hear the warning bells and take notice of what your body is trying to tell you, because your adrenals are most likely shot and you could be heading for a breakdown.

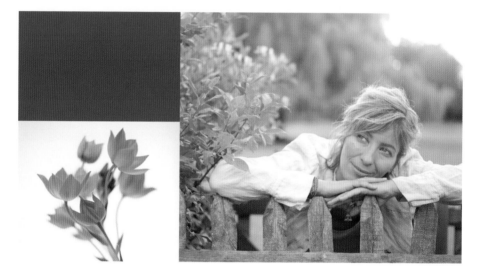

The sad thing is that most of us will recognize at least some of those symptoms in ourselves, because modern life is tough on our poor adrenals. Two tiny little glands that sit above our kidneys and weigh just under five grams apiece when they're healthy, they produce adrenalin and cortisol, the stress hormones that are released in a 'fight or flight' situation. For thousands of years these hormones have helped humans find an extra boost of energy to escape from predators, or fight back in dangerous situations. The problem is, though, our body often doesn't know the difference between a man-eating lion and an irate customer, between fighting for your life and battling through a busy shopping centre. We are very rarely in real physical danger, but anything from a work deadline to driving in rush-hour traffic will get our adrenals pumping.

It's time to see that red flag, hear the warning bells and take notice of what your body is trying to tell you.

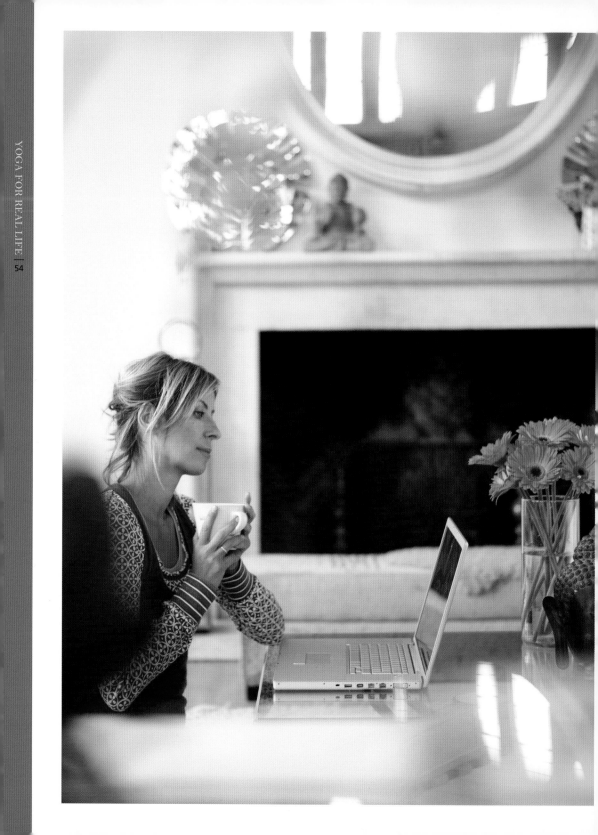

And here's the thing: we get addicted to that adrenalin rush. Sometimes, if we're honest with ourselves, we may even create stressful situations – leaving that report or essay till the last minute, getting distracted by some unimportant task and then not having the time we need to drive to that meeting – because we use the adrenalin to fuel us. The problem is, like most fuel, it eventually runs out. The adrenals can grow up to two grams more as they desperately try to keep up, but eventually they get exhausted, and you slowly start to lose interest in life.

Kundalini yoga and meditation can help enormously with rebuilding strength in the adrenals and coping with stress, and the exercises below will give you back your energy, clarity and zest for life. I was recently contacted by Karen, whose seventy-two-year-old father, Dayton, had started practising Kundalini on the advice of his counsellor. Dayton had suffered from depression for as long as Karen could remember, but she says it was only when she moved in next door to her parents that she realized how bad it was. He worried constantly, was negative about almost everything, and suffered from nightmares that made him afraid to go to sleep. He would start projects but never finish them, which just compounded his stress and depression. Then, two years ago, the stress pushed his blood pressure so high that he suffered a mini-stroke.

Her dad is from a poor farming family in Texas, and not the kind of man who would be naturally drawn to yoga. 'He's not a man of meditation,' laughs

Meditation can help enormously with rebuilding strength and coping with stress.

Karen. 'He's always relied on doctors to tell him what to do.' Since medicines hadn't helped, he agreed to try Kundalini, and after his first set of exercises he went to bed and had his first full, nightmare-free sleep in years. Soon he began to smile more, and although his blood pressure is still high, when it soars to dangerous levels he finds he can bring it down quickly by practising breathing exercises. He does exercises for the adrenals (see page 76) every day, and a longer set of Kundalini movements two or three times a week.

'He still has some medical problems, but for the most part they're much better. And we really believe that it is the yoga that has prevented him having another stroke.'

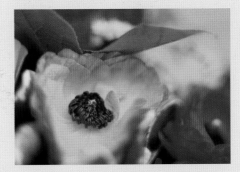

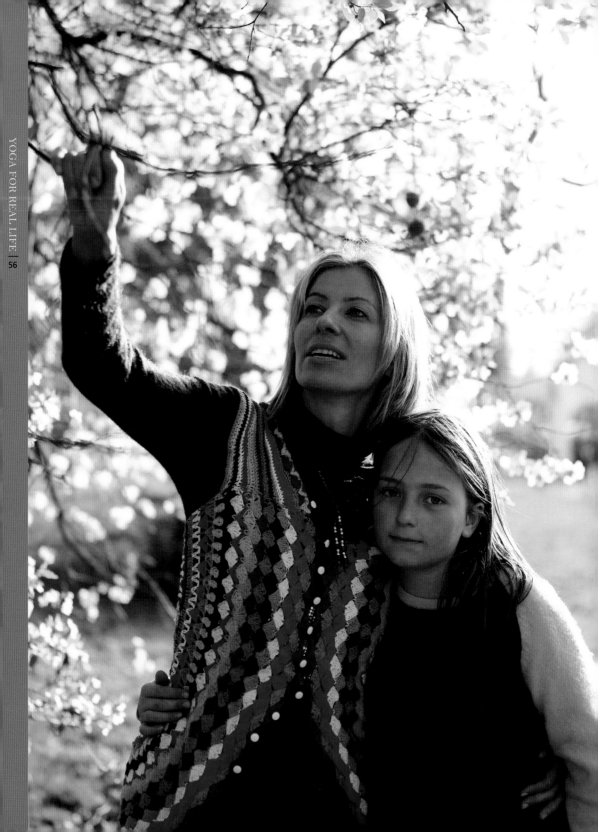

# Making the time

YOU PROBABLY ALREADY HAVE A MANTRA, something you repeat to yourself all day. Since our thoughts, the stories we tell ourselves about the world, help to create our experiences, our mantra shapes our life. We say, 'I'm so tired!' 'I'm really stressed,' 'I don't know what I'm doing,' 'I'm not good enough!' 'It will never happen.' And sure enough, it becomes a self-fulfilling prophecy. We are tired, stressed and unsure, and the things we long for don't happen – mainly because we've talked ourselves out of even trying for them!

'Slow down and enjoy life. It's not only the scenery you miss by going too fast – you also miss the sense of where you are going, and why.'

EDDIE CANTOR (1892–1964)

In the West, one of our most common mantras is 'I don't have time.' If you keep repeating it, one thing is for sure: you won't have time. Think of someone you really admire. Whether it's Bill Gates, Paula Radcliffe, Barack Obama, the Dalai Lama, J. K. Rowling or that other mum you see in the playground, dropping off her three kids calmly before leaving for her high-powered job, looking immaculate, every day, they have the same twenty-four hours as you have – as we all have.

When you wake up, do you take a few minutes to be grateful, to do a few exercises to warm up your spine, and to sit for five minutes, meditate and mentally prepare yourself for the day? No, because you have the kids to see to, you have to rush to work, you need your sleep so you stay in bed for as long as possible. You'll have a thousand reasons, but just try getting up fifteen minutes earlier and giving yourself this little gift. Ask your kids to get their school bags ready by the door before bedtime, lay your work clothes out the night before, go to bed fifteen minutes earlier – do whatever you need to do to create that space for yourself at the very start of your day, and see how much better, how much more calmly that day unfolds. Take those few minutes to plug yourself in to the source, to recharge your batteries, and you will get more done in your day, you'll rush less, and you'll have a clearer idea of what is really important rather than getting tangled up in trivia. You'll *create* more time.

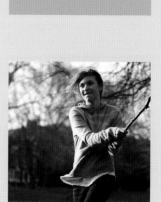

I met Susan at a yoga workshop in London. She had been doing Kundalini for six months. 'I've really noticed that I've stopped rushing around so much,' she said. 'I take more walks in the forest now; I take more time out in general. I have more time for the family, more time for *people*, and it's changed everything for the better. When my friends say they don't have time, I point out that our mums and grandmothers didn't have cars, dishwashers or convenience foods, they had to do the laundry with a mangle, bring up their kids and they often had jobs too. If they had time, why don't we?'

One way of making time is to make your own yantra, a visual of your life. I make mine in the shape of an infinity sign, which looks like a figure 8 tipped on its side. In each of the circles I mark the twelve hours of the clock, one circle for a.m., one for p.m. Next I map out the day, blocking out hours for sleep, work, all the things I need or want to do. For most people, at first it's all pretty much one big block, which is chaos. So we're worshipping the god of chaos rather

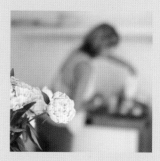

than the goddess of time. It can also be a big shock, as you block in work, chores, looking after the family and everything else you do in a day, to realize just how little time you give yourself! But once you're aware of that, you can start making changes.

If you think you don't have fifteen minutes to do some yoga, meditate or get off the bus to work a few stops early and walk through the park, look at your yantra carefully: you might find you spend three hours a night slumped in front of the TV, that the chores you do after work could be fitted into a lunch-break, that you no longer actually enjoy meeting that friend on Wednesdays for a drink and a gossip and you could suggest going to a yoga class together instead. Twenty-four hours is a long time! You can do a lot in a day, so don't tell me you don't have five minutes. Change your daily mantra. Start saying, 'I have so much time. I have plenty of time.'

# The power of mantra

IN KUNDALINI YOGA, meditation and mantra are used to clear the mind of conscious, ego-driven thoughts that restrict us from experiencing joy. A mantra consists of a series of sounds – often Sanskrit words with powerful meanings – specifically designed for different effects. They can be deceptively simple, such as the 'Wahe guru' chant on page 46. Chanting repetitively clears the negative and stagnated energies that accumulate within us, and while we focus on the sounds we clear our minds more easily of other mental clutter.

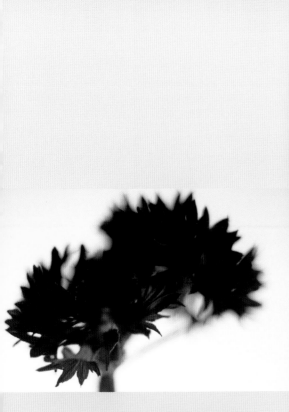

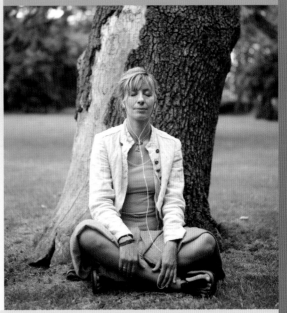

Mantra is a powerful device for effecting change within our bodies by stimulating the immune system. There are an incredible eighty-four reflex points around the mouth that are activated by the vibrations of chanting. These in turn trigger the hypothalamus, a gland in the brain responsible for controlling important metabolic, hormonal and behavioural processes, which then releases naturally occurring opiates called endorphins to stimulate the immune system. As a result we experience a lowering of blood pressure, reduced anxiety and depression and a blissful, peaceful feeling. The kind of breathing chanting encourages is important too, because deep, rhythmic breathing increases oxygen intake and pumps the lymphatic system, our body's sewerage system. A sluggish lymphatic system can lead to health problems over time, including weight gain, muscle loss, high blood pressure, fatigue and inflammation.

It's important to learn exactly how to phrase a mantra to get the desired effect, and if you're feeling unsure, you can hear me chanting all the mantras in this book on my website, www.mayaspace.com. A mantra is repeated over and over again, sometimes for up to thirty minutes. This might sound rather bizarre to the uninitiated, but once you've been in a room with twenty or so people chanting and the energy rises and rises, you will not fail to feel the rush!

Once you begin practising it, the focus and calmness you get while repeating a mantra is something you can access any time you need it. Recently I was hiking up a canyon in California with a friend. I'm fit and I knew I could handle it, but the path was very steep, it was a hot day and I wasn't used to it – I was fighting for breath. So I suggested we stop talking, and just focus and use the hike as meditation. I started repeating the mantra 'Wahe guru' in my head, breathing in and out and timing my steps in rhythm, and as I focused inwards, the tiredness and breathlessness went instantly. I carried on for an hour without any stopping, and it was so easy and flowing. My pulse was very steady and I wasn't even sweating, even though the hill was getting steeper and steeper. When we reached the top, the glorious view over the ocean was well worth it – and my friend had seen the power of mantra for himself. He said it was amazing, that unless he'd seen it with his own eyes, he wouldn't have believed how completely I'd changed.

On another occasion, mantra had an even more dramatic effect. One summer when we were in Greece on a yoga retreat, my husband Magnus persuaded me against my better intuition to accompany him on a swim across a bay to a temple that sat dramatically on a small hill above the rocks about a kilometre away. The sun was about to set and the pinkish early evening glow on the temple pillars was glorious, but having swam less than halfway, we realized we had hit a riptide current that was dragging us out to sea. I started to panic, as my energy was sapping, and I screamed hysterically at Magnus, berating him for having got us into this mess. Then, in the face of all this

Look, I know how weird it seems, because I remember my own reaction when I first went to Kundalini classes. But if you can get past your embarrassment, you'll find it so rewarding.

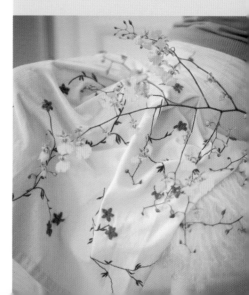

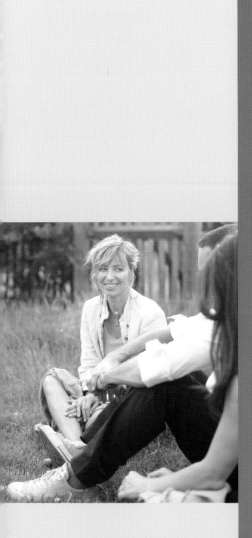

So leave those inhibitions at the door and really open up heart and soul!

fear, I quit fighting and accepted my situation. I began to chant a mantra and almost immediately I found a resource of energy I could not believe was in me. After about an hour we were able to tack across the current and reach the safety of the shore. It had been scary, but mantra saved my life.

By now you may be thinking that whatever the benefits, you're not going to try this one. Look, I know how weird it seems, because I remember my own reaction when I first went to Kundalini classes. But if you can get past your embarrassment, you'll find it so rewarding. Many newcomers to my classes who have never chanted before have to overcome a bit of self-consciousness. It is sad but true that in our culture today, singing out loud and proud is considered a bit odd unless it's either in church, usually a tuneless murmur from a congregation of foot-shufflers, or during a tipsy performance on a karaoke machine at the office party. Overcoming this shyness is an important part of the process. So leave those inhibitions at the door and really open up heart and soul!

Trust me, everyone can sing. Because I'm a musician, people sometimes assume it has been easy for me. But I'm a classically trained pianist, not a singer, and the first time I tried chanting mantra, my voice was so faint it was barely there. But now the pleasure I get from it, from getting that sound out of myself, is enormous. It's pure healing. Chanting is the easiest tool to get you to that stillness. And believe me, I tried everything! Then I realized, chanting is it. Zoom! It just gets me there.

None of the mantras in this book are difficult. Some are monotone, so you only have to pay attention to the words and the sound: it's not really about melody and singing. But it opens your diaphragm, and, without even thinking, you'll find you feel more open, you can breathe better, you can hold the sound easily, for longer. You just have to try it, be open for it. What I've learned, teaching yoga, is that the people who protest most that they can't sing, they won't sing, are the ones who end up enjoying it most. They try a little, and by the third class they're the loudest. I've seen it again and again.

The point of mantra is repetition. Concentrate on it, and after a few minutes your chattering mind will stop screaming, 'This is stupid!' 'I must look mad!' or 'I don't have time for this.' You'll find it harder to dwell on trivial thoughts such as what you need to buy for dinner, or whether you let the cat out. Instead, slowly, you'll feel a sense of infinite space around you.

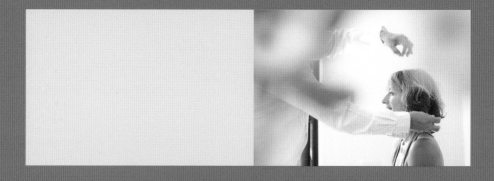

Go deep within. Relax your hands, arms and face. Loosen up your body. You may start to feel you are melting, becoming one with the space around you. There may be a tingling in your hands and toes – this is quite normal.

When you finish, stay quiet and still. Meditate for a minute or two and allow the body, mind and spirit to unite. Listen to any messages or insights that come through, as this is the time you will receive answers to your questions – even ones you didn't know you'd asked! Only you will hear the answers. It's a very personal and precious moment, and a good opportunity to ask for a blessing from your higher power, whatever that may be. It could be God, nature, the Universe, your better self – wherever you believe love, goodness and wisdom come from.

Mantra has become a core part of my daily routine. I really don't know how I'd cope without it. Even my children appreciate that their mother is a lot calmer if she's left in peace to do her daily chant. In fact, they composed their own mantra: *Give her space/ Give her time/ If she does mantra/ She'll be fine.*

Even my children appreciate
that their mother is a lot
calmer if she's left in peace
to do her daily chant.

# Some thoughts on creativity

WE ARE ALL CREATIVE BEINGS, but creativity is something many of us have forgotten how to express. In previous generations, before ready-made food, clothes and furniture were available cheaply in shops, people made their own. We were made to create, not just to consume, and whether baking a cake, telling a story, arranging flowers or seeing shapes in the clouds, everybody has the creative impulse within them. If we perform even the smallest task with imagination, our lives feel richer and more varied.

As you practise the exercises in this chapter, you may start hearing a voice deep within telling you to buy some red shoes and go dancing, to look in a newsagent's window for a flyer advertising pottery or dressmaking classes, to start a journal, buy some watercolours or plant a window-box. Don't dismiss it. Encourage these impulses. Act on them. And when you hear other voices in that endless stream of internal chatter telling you that this is stupid, learn to ignore those thoughts and carry on anyway.

The point here isn't necessarily to write a bestseller or win the Turner Prize, it is to have fun. Start small, and don't expect perfection. And who knows where it may lead?

## Go with the flow

Whatever your passion, go for it. Give it your love and utter dedication, and disciplined focus. *Believe* in your abilities. Inspiration is not an external force, but a flame that burns within. It makes us feel excited, motivated and limitless. Ideas are the seeds from which our creations evolve and grow. And if we commit ourselves to planting and nurturing them, they will eventually bear fruit. We should be prepared to let some wither and fade too, in the knowledge that others more robust will flower and bloom.

The first impulse is normally quite modest, but bit by bit, new elements will come in. Some ideas will be revised and improved and others, however precious, deleted, until something of true substance arises. It's a bit like navigating a fantastic maze: there will be dead ends, and sometimes we may even have to go back to the beginning and start again. The secret is to enjoy the journey as much as attaining the goal.

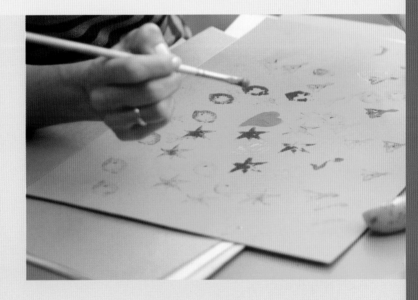

Try to make every moment of your life artistic in some way. Be innovative. Practise routine-breaking. Try wearing a colour you never usually wear, cooking a new dish, rearranging the furniture or painting a wall a bold, bright new shade. Make up songs on car journeys about friends you've just visited, collect stones from the beach and paint faces on them, make your own greeting cards, get your favourite photographs blown up and printed on canvas and hang them on your walls.

# My creative journey

## Music and freedom

As a child in Yugoslavia I wanted to play the piano as far back as I can remember. Whenever we visited my great-aunt Sylvana, I would be drawn to her keyboard and would lose myself in the sound, holding one note and feeling it resonate, then adding other notes until I was drenched in harmony.

Although my parents tried to convince me that a violin would be a more practical and cheaper option, they finally relented and at the age of six I was enrolled at the Skopje Music School. From then I sensed purpose in my life. I would practise three to four hours a day after school. I was very shy as a child and wouldn't talk much. All my emotional expression came through music.

By 1990 I had settled on a career as a concert pianist. Yugoslavia had been dissolved and Macedonia had just become independent. But it was still rife with political unrest and ethnic tensions that would eventually give way to war, and years of Communism had left the people worn and compliant, with a blinkered perspective. So when I moved to London I was filled with excitement. The city seemed impossibly big, with every layer of life you could imagine. The eighties were over and recession was in the air, but in the circles I moved in it seemed glamour was still on the menu. If I was to make it anywhere, I felt, this was the place.

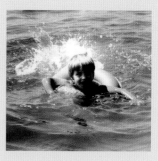

## Finding success, losing the joy

At that time, when London was less international than it is now, I was considered rather exotic. I'd naively accept invitations to glitzy parties and restaurants where I would entertain the celebrity crowd with the fastest and most crowd-pleasing pieces. This got me noticed, and I soon found myself playing to more prestigious audiences. I quickly sussed out that I could achieve more from networking than from months of touring the backwaters of England. I was quite ruthless in many ways, and saw my influential acquaintances only as stepping-stones.

Although my piano technique was continually improving, I began to feel my heart wasn't in it. The piano had filled my childhood with joy and purpose, but the more I used it as a means for achieving success, the more I felt disconnected from it. The more I struggled to fulfil my dreams of fame, deep inside the less inclined I was to be that person, creating a blockage that kept me from my once clear goal. Although on the outside I was still the life and soul of the party, inside my suppressed spirit was crying out.

## Time for a change

I had been classically trained to play only the notes on the page in front of me. So when Ed, a friend and fellow musician, suggested that I try writing my own music, the idea seemed crazy and forbidden.

He showed me how to extemporize from an existing piece, starting with a Mozart piano concerto. I started playing from the first page of the score, and then he pulled it away. 'Don't stop,' he shouted, so I played on but this time I took the music where my heart felt it should go.

Although I was exhilarated by this experience, I was also unsure.

Creating something from scratch? Where would I start?

How would I find the time and inspiration?

What if it wasn't any good?

### Set your spirit free

Next time Ed and I met, I played him an improvisation based on a Macedonian folk song, and he encouraged me to continue working on it. Over the next few weeks I continued to bring him ideas and sketches, which he would help me arrange into full-blown pieces. When I saw what a seed of an idea could become in capable hands, I was motivated. I would sit at the piano, close my eyes and hold my hands over the keyboard. After a few seconds, as if from nowhere, the notes would come. I felt as if I had opened a secret door that had been locked for years and now sunlight was streaming in. My creative instincts were energized and a feeling of joy overcame me, a feeling no material success had given me.

I realize now that for years I had hidden behind a self-projected idea of myself, which kept my true spirit under lock and key. We need to shift a lot of conditioning before we can tap into our true potential. When the mind/ego gets in the way and our motivation is wrong, we will often find a blockage in the flow.

The first time I had played my own compositions in public, I was a bag of nerves. The first half went smoothly – I rattled off a programme of classical pieces that were predictable crowd-pleasers, although I didn't set the night on fire – and then, after the interval, I took the stage to play my own compositions. I had an amazing line-up of talented players behind me, which gave me a real confidence boost. But I was astonished at the roar of approval that greeted the end of the first piece. The blend of cinematic piano, ethnic rhythms, Macedonian folk and virtuoso playing seemed to have hit the mark. They liked it!

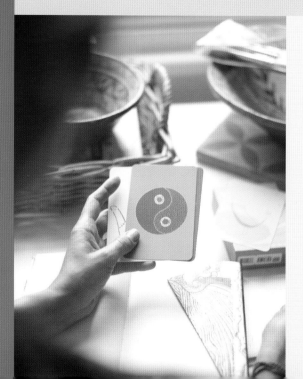

We were made to create, not just to consume, and whether baking a cake, telling a story, arranging flowers or seeing shapes in the clouds, everybody has the creative impulse within them. If we perform even the smallest task with imagination, our lives feel richer and more varied.

## Venus Dream

Peaches are often considered symbolic of sexuality and sensuality. This drink is orange, the colour traditionally associated with the second chakra, and it will inspire your senses and heal your body.

2 or 3 small peaches, cut into chunks
240ml (1 cup) almond milk, or plain yoghurt
    thinned with water
$1/2$ teaspoon chopped fresh mint leaves
$1/2$ teaspoon ground cardamom
1 teaspoon finely chopped fresh ginger
honey to taste

Put all the ingredients into a blender and purée. Serve with passion and love.

## Adrenals

These exercises balance and rejuvenate the adrenals and build back strength if you're feeling tired, unfocused, or close to burnout.

Sit cross-legged in Easy Pose (see page 18), and interlace your little fingers in front of your solar plexus, with your thumbs up. Now pull your fingers in opposite directions and start the Breath of Fire (see below and page 103), breathing in and out hard and loudly through the nose, really pumping the breath from your belly. You will feel a pull across the back. Do this for one to three minutes. This pose will generate heat, and works on the left side of the adrenals.

Still in Easy Pose, follow with Cannon Breath (see below), relaxing your hands in your lap and breathing loudly through the mouth. Again, repeat for one to three minutes. This strengthens the right side of the adrenals.

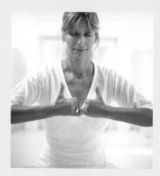

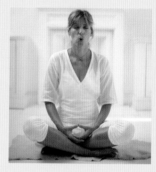

## Breath of Fire

Rapidly inhale and exhale through both nostrils, just like sniffing; it is the best detoxifying breath.

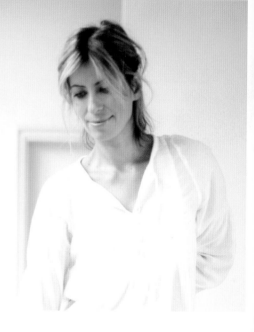

## Cannon Breath

Pucker your mouth into a firm O shape. Now breathe through the mouth loudly, keeping your inhale and exhale equal, as in the Breath of Fire. The name Cannon Breath comes from the sound your breath should make.

## Bridge Pose

This challenging posture tones the spine and strengthens the reproductive organs and kidneys. It stimulates the hormones to secrete and helps to relieve various gynaecological disorders.

Sit with your legs stretched out in front of you and place your hands firmly on the floor behind you. Breathe in and lift the buttocks up, feet flat to the floor and knees bent, supporting yourself with your hands so that the body is parallel to the ground. Let your head fall back. Continue breathing normally for up to two minutes. Apply the Root Lock (see page 19), squeezing your anus and navel in. Then relax and lie down on your back for up to a minute.

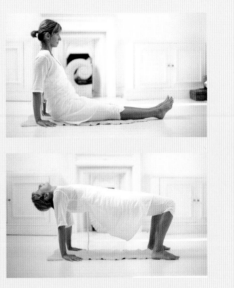

## Alternative: Pelvic Lift

This is a variation on the Bridge Pose that is slightly easier.

Lie on your back with your knees bent, your heels touching your buttocks. As you inhale, hold the ankles and lift the pelvis up. Exhale and come down. After one to three minutes, relax for at least thirty seconds.

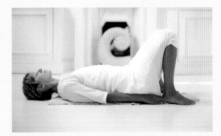

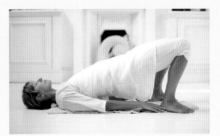

## Flow

This will help you take a more flexible approach to things, to go with the flow rather than fighting it all the time. It is great for bringing inspiration into your life, and it will open you to the abundance all around you. It's a great one to try if you're experiencing money worries!

Lie on your stomach with your forehead on the floor. Interlace your fingers behind your back in Venus Lock (see page 72). Lift your legs and arms, keeping your knees and elbows as straight as possible, and start the Breath of Fire (see page 76), breathing in and out through your nose noisily and rapidly. Tense your buttocks to protect your lower back.

If you find lifting your legs challenging, keep them on the floor. This exercise will stimulate flow in your life so that you find everything you do easier.

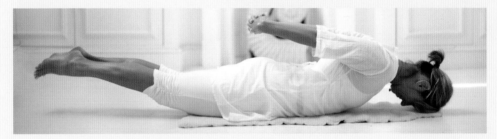

## Body Drops

This position puts pressure on the kidneys and flushes toxins. It gives you more energy, waking up the Kundalini, and will make you stronger, both physically and mentally. Do it just twice a week, and you'll see results.

Sit in Easy Pose (see page 18), or with your legs straight out in front of you – whichever feels most comfortable. Make your hands into fists, then start lifting your buttocks by pushing your fists into the ground and dropping down on to your sitting bones. If that is too uncomfortable for your hands, lay your palms flat on the floor instead of making fists, and push from there. Inhale as you go up, and exhale as you come down. Continue for one to three minutes.

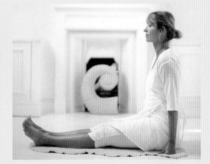

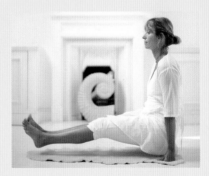

## Sat Kriya

This deceptively simple, self-contained exercise is the most powerful in the science of Kundalini yoga. It stimulates circulation, balances energy, perfects the functioning of the sex organs and works on the 72,000 nerves in the navel area, which in turn triggers the rising of the Kundalini energy. It opens the channel of creativity. If you want to bring more creativity into your life, this is the one to try.

Sit on your heels, or if you find that too difficult sit cross-legged in Easy Pose (see page 18) or on a chair. Stretch your arms above your head, touching your ears, with hands clasped together and index fingers pointing up. Close your eyes and focus your attention on the third eye, the invisible point midway between your eyebrows, in order to stimulate the pituitary gland and open your vision and intuition. Remember to drop your shoulders and keep them relaxed even when the arms are up, to avoid tension.

Chant 'Sat!' loudly and sharply while pulling your navel in with a rapid, jerking movement. Imagine someone punching you in the stomach. Then chant a longer, softer 'Nam' (*naaaaaam*) as you release your navel. The breath will come automatically. Repeat for as long as you can. Start with one to three minutes, and extend the time as you get more used to it.

On the last exhale, hold the breath and apply the Root Lock (see page 19), pulling in your navel, anus and sex organs as hard as you can. Hold for a few seconds, and release. When you are finished, lie down in Corpse Pose (see page19) and relax.

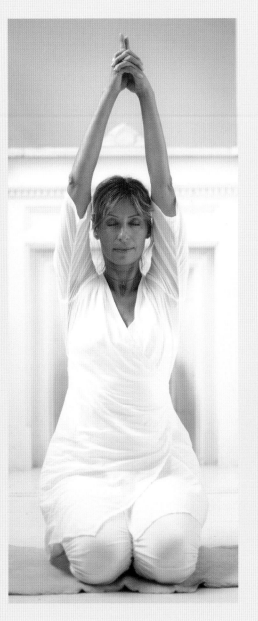

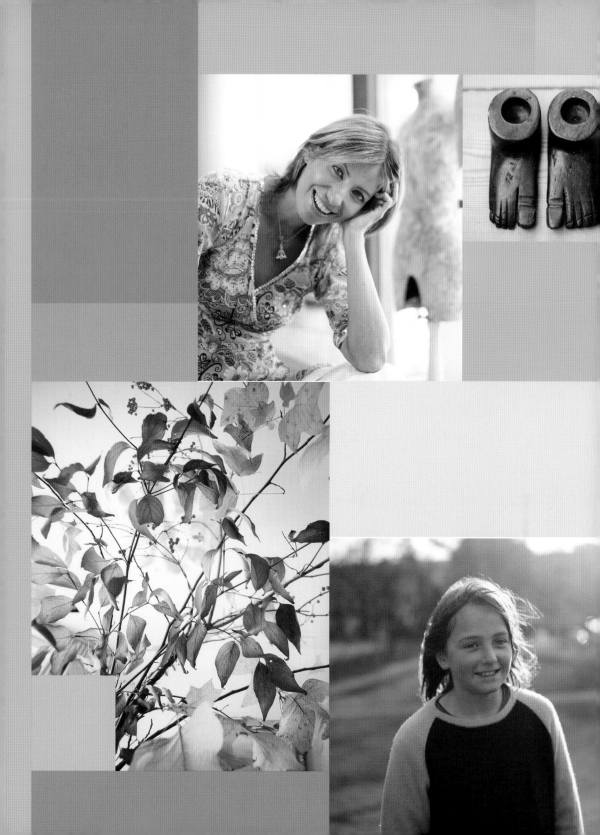

# Yes, I Can!

# NAVEL CHAKRA

THE THIRD CHAKRA IS IN THE STOMACH AREA and affects the digestive system, liver, gall bladder, spleen and pancreas. If you are blocked or unbalanced in this area, it can cause eating disorders, digestive problems and low energy levels as well as negative emotions such as anger, greed, envy, shame and despair. It's also the area to work on if you are having problems with diet and digestion – including over-eating. It's no coincidence that very few Kundalini practitioners suffer from Irritable Bowel Syndrome.

If you're stressed or nervous, you feel it in your stomach. It's where you also sense your intuition – literally, your gut feelings. This chakra affects your self-esteem, power, willpower – it's where that feeling of 'Yes, I can!' comes from. It's the centre for personal power. Are you a 'doer', exuberant and expressive? Can you initiate and complete an action? How you project and manifest anything in your life depends on balance in this area. The person who is centred in this chakra achieves every action and will inspire others in order to do so.

| GOVERNS: | SHADOW | COLOUR: | SYMBOL: | ELEMENT: |
|---|---|---|---|---|
| Courage, self-esteem, willpower: the energy and commitment needed to take action and see it through | EMOTIONS: Anger, greed and envy | Yellow | A lotus with ten petals | Fire |

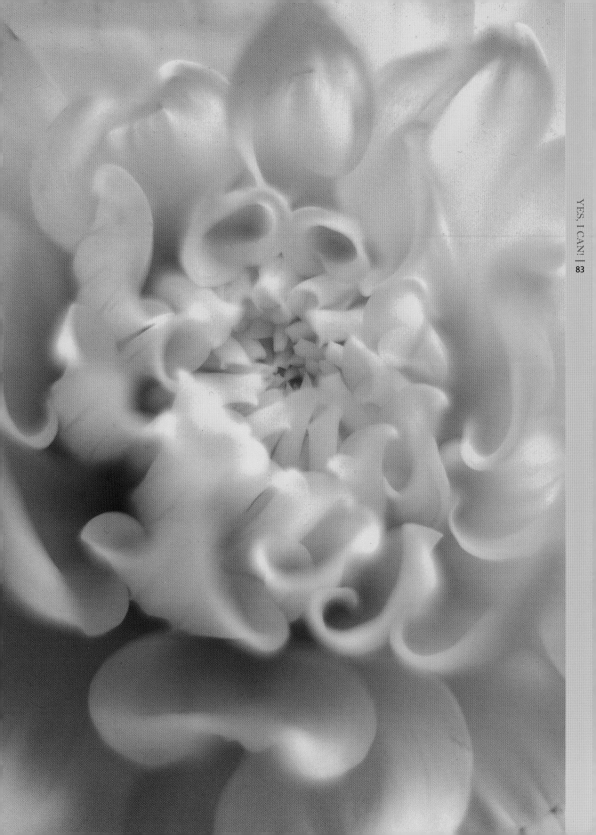

# Building confidence

WITH THE EXERCISES IN THE FIRST CHAKRA, WE WERE LAYING NEW FOUNDATIONS. In the second, we learned how to flow and go with changes. Now it's all about action.

Confidence comes from within, but also from doing, keeping your word to yourself, resolving to do something and following through. As you practise Kundalini, for instance, you notice that every day you're getting stronger, you can hold the positions for longer. It doesn't matter if you're wobbly at first, if you struggle, if I suggest you repeat something for three minutes and you're exhausted after one. What matters is that you try again a minute later, or next day, and the day after that. That you focus and believe, until one day – sooner than you'll think – you'll realize you are doing it effortlessly.

Kellie found one of my Kundalini DVDs at her local library. She'd had three babies in three years, her father had died and she'd turned to food to give her the comfort she needed to cope. She was tired, she felt numb, and she weighed 218lb. It took her weeks to play the DVD, and the first time she followed it, she struggled to even sit on the floor.

> 'If I have lost confidence in myself, I have the universe against me.'
>
> RALPH WALDO EMERSON
> (1803–82)

'Easy Pose wasn't easy for me!' she laughs. 'After twenty minutes, I was panting and had to stop – I couldn't believe that was just the warm-ups.' But here's the key: she persevered. Next time she sat on a folded towel to make it easier, and within a few sessions she found she could do without it, and was able to follow the routine to the end. 'That gave me confidence to carry on, and soon in yoga I'd found the peace I'd been praying for. I feel so light on my feet after every session, I feel like dancing – a big difference from my life before! I felt so energized and inspired, I started looking forward to it. I didn't ever put myself on a diet. I lowered my portion sizes, and began to want healthier foods. Eventually, as a family, we decided to go vegetarian, because it just felt right for us. And the weight began to fall away.'

Kellie had lost more than 50lb when we spoke, but that wasn't the most important change in her. She felt more positive, more confident. She'd stopped watching violent TV shows. She was reading and studying and following new interests. Her family now goes on regular bike rides together, and Kellie is full of plans for the future.

So just make a decision: yes, I can. Transform the nagging, insistent 'no' in your life into a loud, positive 'yes'. Rather than, 'Oh, I can't!' try saying, 'Why not?' Whatever it is.

When you release this chakra, every day you get stronger and your vision becomes clearer. When you believe in yourself, you can do anything you want to do. It's time to start really focusing on your dreams, your desires, to be positive about what you want in your life.

# Criticism, judgement and envy

'Our envy of others devours us most of all.'
ALEXANDER SOLZHENITSYN (1918–2008)

YOU ARE REALLY STUPID. You're wasting your time reading this book. It's pointless. People will laugh. Anyway, you always mess things up. You're too old. Too ugly. Too fat, too unfit, too weak. You're not good enough. You'll never make anything of your life. You'll never be happy. No one likes you. And did I mention that you're stupid?

Are you offended yet? Perhaps you're starting to think, 'No one talks to me that way!' But the chances are that someone does, and that someone is you. We all have a chorus of inner critics chattering away inside us, little gremlins warning us that everything we do will turn to dust. Listen carefully and you'll hear your own angry voice in there, and also the voices of parents, teachers, ex-partners, all raised in a chorus of disapproval. But just because they are there, it doesn't mean you have to listen to them, or agree with them. You certainly shouldn't let them stop you doing what you want to do.

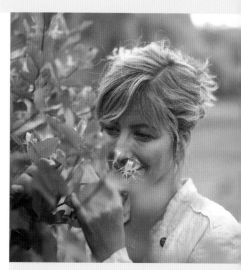

They're just thoughts, and with practice you really don't have to engage with them much at all.

Once you're clear, really enjoy this thing in your head. Use all your senses to bring it to life. Smell the leather seats in that new car; taste that cold beer on the beach; walk through your dream house imagining every room. If there's anything you can do to make it more real, do it – order travel brochures, test-drive your dream car, hang out in the area where you'd like to live.

And then – this is the hard bit – let go of it. Acknowledge that though it would be fun to have this, your life is complete, right now, without it. You don't have to have it. You can be perfectly content without it. The important part is to not get too attached to the outcome. You can achieve anything, but it's all about how you achieve it. Are you going to get stressed about doing it? Or are you just going to say, 'Look, I absolutely believe I can achieve this, I would like it for myself, I would enjoy it, it would be fun, but whatever happens, I'll be OK.' If you can work with that idea, life will be so much easier.

Then be alert for coincidences, little acts of synchronicity that may be the Universe trying to give you what you've asked for. Listen to your own little bursts of inspiration, and act on them. But don't push. Just trust that if it was meant to be, it will come to you in some form or other. Perhaps you'll get your holiday by winning it in a competition. Perhaps you'll realize you can afford to save a sum each month that will get you there in a year or two. Perhaps you'll find a house swap there, or hear about a summer job.

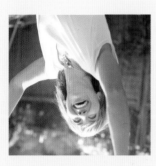

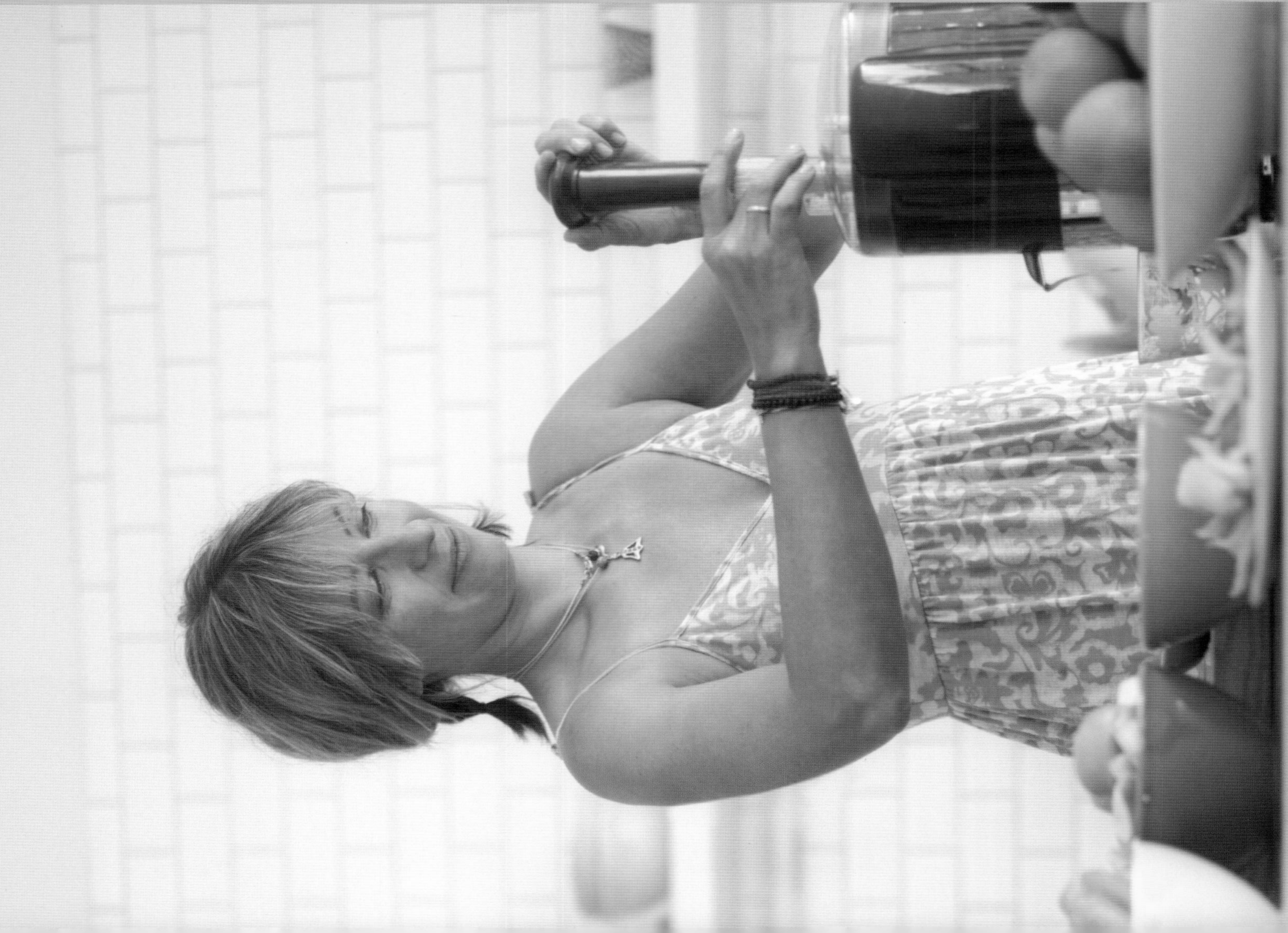

# Love &
# Relationships

# HEART CHAKRA

THE FOURTH CHAKRA, THE HEART CENTRE OF THE BODY, lies in the area of the sternum. It's the place where 'me' becomes 'we'. All the me, me, me – the work you've done on yourself in the first three chakras – is transformed here into 'us' – into sharing, doing it together, into community. This energy point relates to love, compassion, personal expansion and the ability to love selflessly.

This centre doesn't just govern sexual relationships, but our relationships at work, with our kids, with mother nature, everything. When our energy flows through it, the heart is opened and true love becomes possible. If it is out of balance and blocked, we don't feel love. Through Kundalini yoga we can help restore the energy flow and maintain balance. And when we put our heart into something, anything is possible!

GOVERNS:
Compassion, love

SHADOW EMOTIONS:
Fear, rejection and attachment

COLOUR:
Green

SYMBOL:
A lotus with twelve petals

ELEMENT:
Air

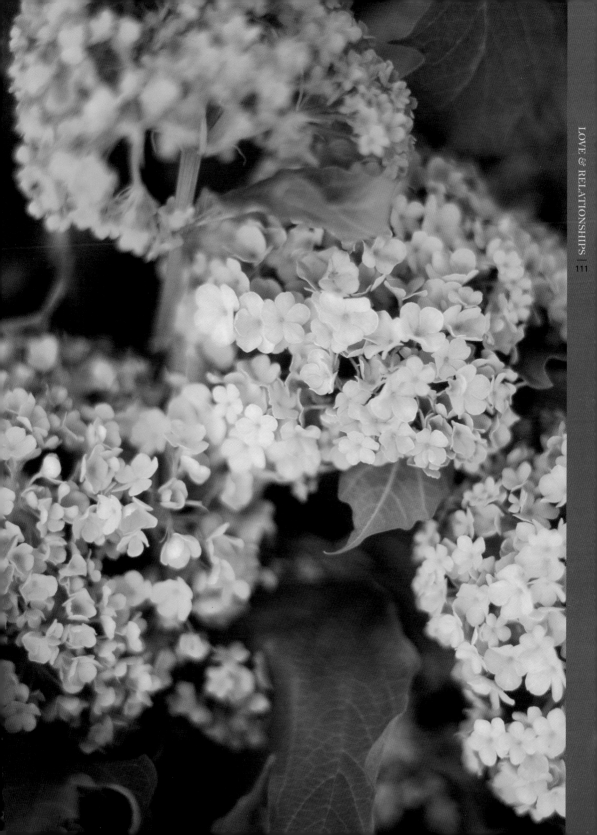

# All you need is love

LET'S START WITH THE MOST IMPORTANT PERSON: YOU. Before you can love anyone or anything else fully, you have to learn to love yourself. How can we share what we don't give ourselves? If you increase how secure and loving you feel about yourself on the inside, you will attract more happiness and love from the outside. You need to relate to yourself authentically, from your heart and soul, before genuinely fulfilling relationships will be possible.

'Your task is not to seek for love, but merely to seek and find all the barriers within yourself that you have built against it.'
RUMI (1207–73)

It is not selfish to love and understand yourself first – it is a gift for your partner to be with someone who is happy and at peace. It's so important. If you forgive yourself and love yourself unconditionally, many other problems disappear. So in the exercises here, we do lots of opening movements. We're saying, 'I love myself. I share myself with others. I offer forgiveness.'

So how do we get to this place of loving and understanding ourselves? One area that often needs to be worked on, especially for women, is how we feel about ourselves sexually. From an early age, women are conditioned to look and act a certain way – to please people – in order to deserve sexual interest from men. It is up to us to lose the expectations that have been foisted upon us, to clear these internalized distortions. We need to start practising self-acceptance and re-evaluating the way we see ourselves.

Sexual confidence is not about having a great body – it's about getting to know your own unique body intimately, celebrating it and finding out what makes you feel good.

When she told me the story she shared on page 85, Kellie explained that she is a photographer by profession. As she grew bigger after having her three children, she made sure she was always behind the camera, not in front, because she knew she would hate what she saw. The turning point came when she made the decision to start loving herself just the way she was. She took her professional camera along with her on a family picnic, and the whole family took turns taking pictures. Later she chose 150 of them to print out, then framed them and put them all over the house. 'When I'm working professionally, I will retouch pictures, get rid of the flaws. But I deliberately left these just as they were, and I loved them. I looked so happy, and so free because I wasn't embarrassed about myself any more.' Soon after this she discovered Kundalini, and the weight began to fall away. But it started with loving herself just as she was, at that moment.

Remember that so-called perfect bodies are few and far between. We feel we have to measure ourselves against the glamorous images in magazines, but the women in these pictures have spent hours having their hair and make-up done, they've been lit in the most flattering way, and that dress is often hanging so perfectly because the back is a mass of pins. They rarely look this perfect in their day-to-day lives. A photographer or magazine designer can make blemishes or wrinkles disappear with the click of a mouse, they can stretch legs longer, nip in a waist, give breasts a few more cup sizes, thicken and shine hair. Often we're measuring ourselves against women who only exist on a computer screen. And astonishingly, even the most conventionally beautiful women often fail to see themselves as they really are. Ask any supermodel or glamorous actress what she would like to improve, and you'll always get a long list of real or perceived flaws!

Learn to focus on the positive. Look good for yourself. Do your Kundalini and your inner and outer beauty will merge in radiant health. But don't wait for that.

Stop judging yourself *now*, and decide not to worry what others think of you. There may be things you want to work on, but try to see that you don't need fixing because you're not broken. Right now, you're perfect just the way you are.

There's nothing more attractive than someone who is comfortable in her own skin, who sees the beauty in herself and looks for the beauty in others rather than judging and criticizing. Walking into a room, the sexually confident woman is relaxed and smiling, so smile and *feel* sexy! When we feel sexy in ourselves, our minds shift from anxious to welcoming. Sexual confidence is about attitude, even power – the power that comes from liking yourself.

You don't need fixing because you're not broken. Right now you're perfect just the way you are.

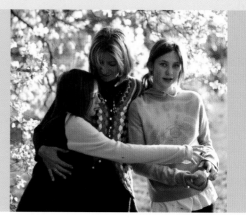

Loving yourself also entails finding out what makes you happy in other areas of life, and going for it! Exercising the heart chakra keeps you open to the instincts and promptings of your heart. Don't live in the past with its old habits – be present in the now, which is where the answers to your questions lie.

We are particularly mean when it comes to treats, feeling we somehow don't deserve them. It might help to keep a list of things you really love: try to add a few every week until you reach at least 100. How many of these do you do on a regular basis? Some, of course,

you can't do all the time, but the world is full of little pleasures that are inexpensive, or even free: going for a walk, watching a good comedy, having a long soak in a hot bath, lighting a scented candle, dancing round the living room to music you love, chatting on the phone to a friend, eating juicy strawberries, buying fresh flowers. Nurturing yourself – whether it's a weekly massage or doing your daily yoga – is a necessity not only for your personal evolution but also to be able to nurture others too. It builds a solid foundation for every relationship in life.

> 'The weak can never forgive. Forgiveness is the attribute of the strong.'
> MAHATMA GANDHI
> (1869–1948)

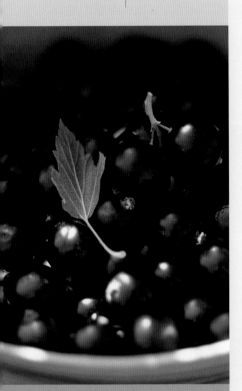

# Spreading the love

TO OPEN YOUR HEART TO LOVE, you need to forgive yourself for your mistakes, for the past, for being judgemental. Then you need to forgive others. Let go of grudges, of anger, and just forgive. Learn to appreciate others, to lavish praise on their achievements rather than constantly pointing out their mistakes. We create our own reality: everything starts with our thoughts, attitudes, reactions. The more you wish others well, the more that same wish comes back to you. It takes a while to grasp this, but once you do, it makes life so much easier and more pleasurable. Keep saying it to people, and you're also saying it to yourself: 'You've no idea how beautiful you are, how wonderful. I appreciate what you do, I'm proud of you!'

Seek out the good in other people, and you'll soon start to see it in yourself. People say, 'I'm not going to have any relationships until I sort myself out,' but the best way to sort yourself out is through relationships! So just be aware of how you react to people, what you wish for them. It's not easy at first, but start with small steps. With all relationships, the trick is not to focus your attention on the other person, to try to change them. Instead focus on yourself, and change your attitude towards them.

## Good Vibrations

Every thought has a vibration, and it's like a ripple effect. If there is a person at work who really annoys you, for instance, next time you see them look at them, and try sending them love. Even if you don't mean it, just say it in your head. In your thoughts, tell them they're smart and beautiful. Wish them all the best. Or just visualize them in a ball of light. Send it to them and surround them with it. It only takes a second. Then see if that person changes towards you. Next time you see them, they might smile at you. And even if they don't respond, after a while you'll find that they no longer annoy you, that you can feel genuine compassion for their behaviour rather than annoyance – but at least you won't let it ruin your day.

It's like a boomerang effect: whatever you wish for them, you wish for yourself. We can all create abundance around us, but it's not just about asking, dreaming, praying. We have to believe in it, we have to be open. We have to allow things to happen to us. And that comes from opening the heart.

Instead of arguing with people, just send them love. And something will happen. Or maybe it won't, but at least you won't let it ruin your day.

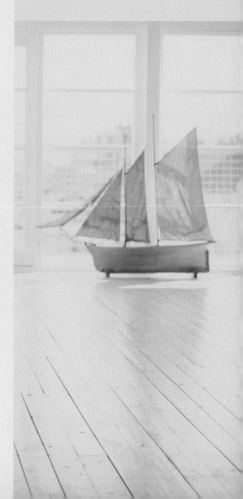

# Friendship

WHEN I FIRST MOVED TO LONDON FROM MACEDONIA, my English was limited and I had no family or friends to rely on. I studied piano in the evenings, but started modelling in the daytime to supplement my income. I met Camilla, who became my flatmate and closest friend, on a modelling assignment at an impossibly smart hotel where the 'ladies who lunch' would assemble to watch us prowl down a catwalk, draped in clothes that were more expensive than my mother's apartment in Skopje. Camilla is a Swedish beauty with an addictive smile and unshakeably calm temperament, the perfect balance for my sometimes hot-tempered Macedonian manner, and we've been friends now for more than twenty years.

'Do not protect yourself by a fence, but rather by your friends.'
CZECH PROVERB

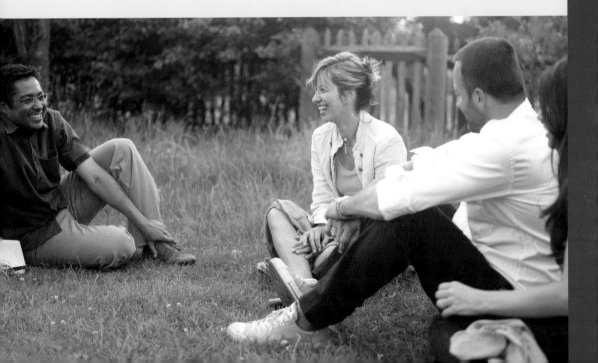

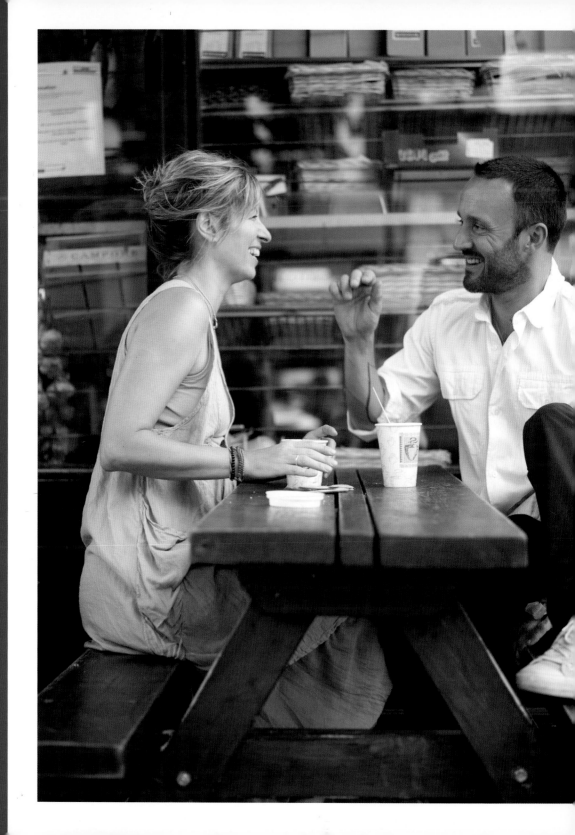

## With a little help from my friends

This kind of genuine friendship – deep, abiding – is one of the most valuable of all forms of relationship. A friend who has been there throughout the changes in your life, witnessed your ups and downs, weathered your highs and lows, and has never wavered in love and support – a friend like this is a priceless gift. People may come and go in our lives, but with some we share a deep connection and bond. We know their support is constant and unconditional. And just as they are there for us, so we are there for them.

When our heart centres are open and energy flows between two friends, we feel the spark of a kindred spirit. Women more often seek out this type of close friendship – we feel the need to find others with whom we can be completely

> When you connect with someone on a level of deep trust, you have created a support system, a place of safety – and someone to have fun with, too!

authentic, with whom we can communicate in confidence: share our secrets, even our shame and our fears. They provide validation and are one of our front-line defences during difficult periods. When you connect with someone on a level of deep trust, you have created a support system, a place of safety – and someone to have fun with, too! Life changes and friendships evolve, but the friend who is genuine is a constant in your life.

## Soul sister, soul brother

Our world is, in a sense, framed by the friends we choose. No friend will ever be completely perfect, but then of course neither are we! However, sometimes we find ourselves with a friend who takes from us without giving back, who depletes our energy and holds us back

from fulfilling our potential. Avoid negative energy, and when your instincts prompt you to pull back from a particular friendship, follow your heart and do so.

As you follow a path of increasing awareness, you may realize that some of your old friends don't suit you any more – they may seem petty, or superficial. One of my students asked me about this recently. She was worried because she didn't want to go out drinking with her friends any more, or to waste time talking about rubbish. But when you're growing, that's what happens: it's like shedding an old skin. Sometimes it's just temporary, while you make your transition. While you're still learning, you're so excited by the changes in yourself you want to shake people and say, 'Look! There is another way!'

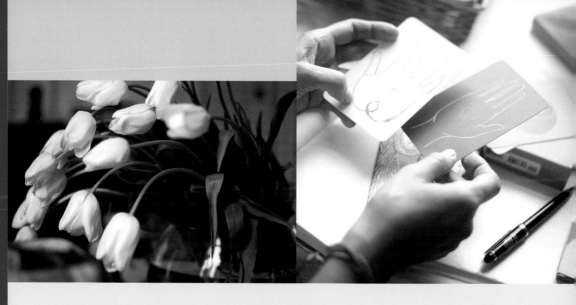

So you go preaching to everyone, and they think, 'Oh, she's gone a bit weird.' Suddenly you don't seem fit in with your old friends. But keep up your yoga and meditation, and you'll get to a point where you no longer feel you have to preach. You're calm, more content. You don't try to convince people of anything, yet they start saying, 'You look great! What have you been doing?' And when you tell them, some of them will say, 'Oh, I want that!'

While you're making changes in your life, it's great to be with people who are on the same level as you, going through the same transition. That's why classes, workshops and yoga holidays work so well. When people come on my yoga retreats, they become friends very quickly – they're strangers, from different backgrounds, but they're going through the same journey.

It's good to have a friend you can talk to. If you're studying the same things or reading the same book, you can talk it over and ask each other questions so you

know you're not losing your mind! But if you have to go it alone, so be it. Your new interests will lead you to new friends. Of course there will be times when you feel, 'I don't want to carry on, this is crazy. I'm really lonely.' But you just have to cry it out and stay with it, because it will change. Those moments are like a test. In the beginning it's exciting, you're meeting new people, but then there will be a drop, a checking point when you have to decide whether to carry on. It's like in the film *The Matrix* – are you going to take the blue pill, or the red pill? Are you going to stay where you are, or move on and grow?

The close friendships we've been discussing don't come along every day. But when your heart is open and the heart chakra is active through Kundalini, you will be able to recognize and welcome the possibilities of these new, deeper connections. You will be able to trust the promptings of your heart and recognize a new soul-sister or soul-brother!

# Sex, love and staying together

CHALLENGES WILL ARISE IN ANY RELATIONSHIP, but especially a long-term union such as marriage. Indeed, marriage is known as the highest – and most difficult – form of yoga! Over time we tend to mirror the best and worst in each other as the relationship evolves, but steady Kundalini practice can find and maintain the point of balance, keeping the lines of communication open.

I met my husband Magnus in 1995, and we were married a few months later. I had been married before, and throughout my twenties I had dipped in and out of relationships, trying to find ways of relating to men. My father had died when I was twelve, so it was difficult for me. I'm also quite individual and independent, and for a long time I felt things had to be my way or no way when it came to relationships. My mother was exactly the same. But I've been learning not be so direct, and it definitely works better.

It's all about balance. Before, I was quite aggressive, quite masculine. And I have to say, some men love that! Then it occurred to me that I was taking on the role of the mother, constantly telling men what to do. I could never stand to see a woman being put down. I'd be the one saying, 'Don't talk to her like that!' I was such a fighter. And I'd say to my friends, 'Are you crazy? Letting him talk to you like that!' But I finally realized you can't change people. You can be there for them, but they need to go through that process, that learning, themselves. As I began to be awakened more with yoga, I started exploring, experimenting with different ways to be more feminine.

Of course there are always things you'd like to change in your partner, but how we feel is not necessarily how they feel. Magnus is a musician and composer, and in the beginning, when I was at home with the kids and he was working long hours in the studio, it wasn't easy for me. But the more forceful I was, the more he would back off – and he'd work even later, because when he did come home, I'd shout at him. Then I realized I needed to work on myself instead. That's when I went deeply into yoga. I was calmer, and Magnus would say, 'This is great, keep going! You're not shouting so much.'

We all take things from our parents, and my mother was like that with my father. So I was projecting their dynamic, without realizing it. Sometimes it's not even your life you're reacting to, it's your parents' life. Again, meditation helps you see those patterns and break free of them.

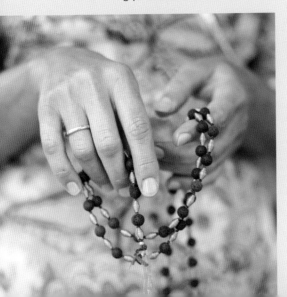

I think Magnus came to realize that he had to put more effort in. And I realized that in a way, I was asking him to change the very thing that attracted me to him in the first place – his passion for music, and his work.

As Kahlil Gibran says in *The Prophet*, space is important in a long-term relationship. I'm sure one of the reasons ours has worked for so long is because we spend so much time apart! If you're happy and content within yourself, it's easier to allow your partner time to pursue their own interests with their own friends. Give each other that trust and freedom, and you'll have new things to share when you are together again.

When you are together, however, try to take time to really *be* together. Even if it's only ten minutes in a busy day, make the effort to focus solely on your partner. Don't talk about bills, the kids or work. Don't bustle about the kitchen while you're talking. Sit down, look them in the eye, take time to really listen to what they're saying. Women especially – we just want to tell them all our troubles, and how our day has gone. We just want to offload, and we sometimes forget to listen. You have to acknowledge each other and respect each other. Always think what you'd want done to you.

Another challenge over a long period of time is to maintain the sense of joy and excitement in your sex life. Yogi Bhajan says, 'Sex happens in the head.' You think about it, you get excited, and you react physically. Sexual energy is one of the most powerful life energies. If, however, the relationship is based on this aspect alone – simple physical gratification – the

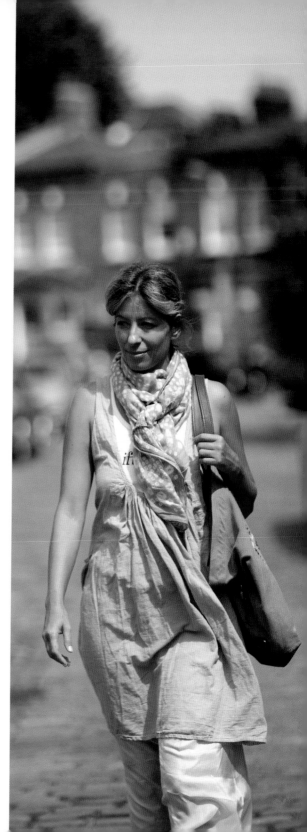

Say how much you love being together, and list all the good things that made you fall in love with each other.

relationship is unlikely to grow into an authentic connection, where the emotional and spiritual needs of the partners are met.

In Kundalini, sexuality is a vehicle to spirituality. It opens up new possibilities for sexual relationships that vibrate in higher frequencies of love, joy and peace. The merging of two souls in joyous sexual pleasure is what we are seeking.

When I work with couples, sometimes I'll put them opposite each other and ask them to just look into each other's eyes, or to touch each other's heart. And many of them can't do it. They're uncomfortable, giggling. Acknowledge your partner, relate to each other, and feel that one-ness. Breathe together, looking into each other's eyes, so you come into the same rhythm and open your heart for the act. Take it slowly! You don't always have to rush.

Sometimes, treat it like a ritual. Prepare the room, light some candles, burn some incense, play calming meditative music in the background, have massage oil handy. Don't rush into it. Take a few long deep breaths together. Give each other compliments – say how much you love being together, and list all the good things that made you fall in love with each other.

Now sit on your heels, touching your partner's knees. Hold each other's hands by interlacing your fingers together in Venus Lock at shoulder level (see page 72). Looking into each other's eyes, pull your navel in as you inhale and very slowly raise your hands. Slowly exhale and bring your hands back down to their original position, releasing your navel. Repeat this action for three minutes. This will generate a strong psycho-magnetic field through which positive energy is channelled, raising your consciousness to a higher divine state. Looking into each other's eyes is a very powerful tool for opening the heart and reminding each other of the times when you used to do that more often – before you became so 'busy' with life.

When you finish, spend some time massaging each other, really experiencing and tuning into the divine energy flowing between you. The rest is your call!

# Being alone…

YOGA FOR REAL LIFE

MOST OF US ARE GOING TO FIND OURSELVES ALONE AT SOME POINT in our lives, whether by conscious choice or as a result of remaining single, being divorced, or losing a loved one. We may be alone for only a specific period of time, such as a self-imposed retreat in order to re-connect with our inner core – or we may remain so indefinitely. In our society it is often assumed that a person alone is to be pitied, or is in some way flawed. Yet in many ways solitude is an empowering and often welcome gift, depending on our particular circumstances.

'In me I have found only one reality: that I breathe in, and I breathe out. And so anything that breathes in or out is reality. When I found this as a reality in everybody, I found myself in everybody and everybody in myself.' YOGI BHAJAN (1929–2004)

It can be a chance to explore our own needs and desires away from the pressures of putting others first, and an opportunity to really get in touch with the area of the fourth chakra that relates to personal growth. If we embrace solitude as an enriching, possibly life-changing experience, we can turn being alone into a time of positive growth. Many of us look outside ourselves for reassurance – from society, our culture, our peers – but the answer most often lies within. Time alone gives us the space to reflect and communicate with ourselves. When we are contemplating change of any kind, for example, some time alone allows us to listen to our heart more clearly.

Meditation is a valuable way of directing our energies towards these possibilities and towards wholeness. We can meditate on our dreams, visualizing goals and being at one with the Universe. We can't always find large chunks of time to be alone, but if we try to create some regular time to be by ourselves we will be able to access the stillness that opens us to our essential energy, to pay attention to our instincts and channel this energy to good places. There are many different ways to find time for yourself – even something as simple as a long, hot bath surrounded by candles, getting up early to practise Kundalini, listening to uplifting music, or going for a long drive. The reflective qualities gained from even these relatively shorter periods of alone-time can be extremely valuable.

As we learn through solitude to connect to our deeper and higher selves and become more self-aware, living life more fully and creatively, we find that these gains can enhance our relationships in new, vital ways.

Now, clearly, there is a difference between choosing to spend time alone and having it forced upon us. The pain of divorce or the loss of a loved one and the subsequent loneliness is immeasurable. It is one of the paradoxes of life that if we dare to love, we will often lose it one way or another, and grief is inevitable. Healing takes time, but profound wisdom is often accumulated after loss. We can heal when we turn our pain into something meaningful, and helping others is key to helping ourselves. Practising self-love and self-nurture is now more important than ever. And alone as we feel at these times, we are never really alone.

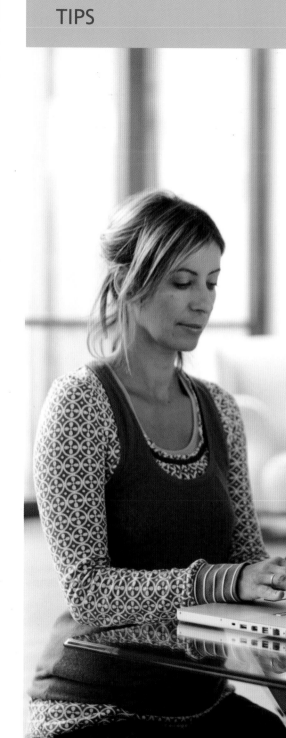

## HOW TO COPE WITH SOMEONE WHO ANNOYS YOU

Let's say it's someone at work, and you know you have a meeting with them that day. Think about that meeting before you get up in the morning. See it happening. Send love to that person. And see him or her smiling back. If they're the kind of person who gets angry, try to feel compassion when you meet. Just say, 'I'm so sorry you're feeling like that.' To do this well, you need to stay calm. Just before the meeting, go to the bathroom, inhale through your nose, then do a powerful, noisy, whistling exhale through your mouth. Do this ten times. You'll be so chilled out you'll be able to cope with the situation calmly.

# RECIPE

## Love Tonic

This delicious red drink will fill your belly with the fire of passion. Hawthorn berries are excellent for cardiovascular health, while hibiscus is high in Vitamin C.

360ml (1 $\frac{1}{2}$ cup) filtered water
5cm piece of fresh root ginger,
     peeled and quartered
2 tablespoons hibiscus flowers
1 $\frac{1}{2}$ teaspoons hawthorn berries
$\frac{1}{2}$ tablespoon rose water
1 $\frac{1}{2}$ teaspoons raw honey or agave syrup

Put the ginger into a pan with the water. Bring to the boil and simmer for 10 minutes. Turn off the heat and add the hibiscus flowers and hawthorn berries. Leave to stand for a minimum of 5 minutes. Stir in the rose water and add honey or agave syrup to sweeten. Serve warm or chilled.

# EXERCISES

### Crisscross Hands (Heart Opener)

This helps to open up your heart, clears grief, and increases forgiveness. It also stimulates the thymus gland, strengthening your immune system.

Sit in Easy Pose (see page 18) and extend both arms up and out, creating a 'V' shape. Keep elbows straight and criss-cross your arms in front of your face. Synchronize your movement with the Breath of Fire (see page 76) for one and a half minutes.

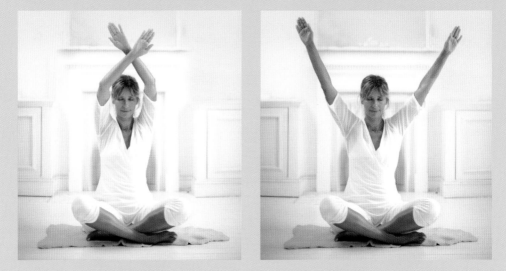

### Venus Triangle

I'm often asked by my students to teach them techniques for dealing with arguments: what to do when we see red and can't help it, when we find ourselves in deep and can't stop the momentum. It may take some doing to persuade your partner to do this with you at that point, but it will stimulate the release of endorphins and make you both feel more positive. You'll forget what you were arguing about and start laughing. It is all ego-driven drama. See the humour in it. Does fighting for your opinion really matter? Ask yourself: do you want to be right, or do you want to be happy?

Stand back to back and about two feet away from your partner. Now each of you do the following. Place your feet hip-width apart. Bend forward with palms touching the ground and shoulder-width apart, and push your hips up to come into the Triangle Pose – also known as Downward Dog – the backs of your heels should be touching your partner's heels. Your weight should be evenly distributed between your feet and hands, your head and neck loose and relaxed as your arms take the strain. Gaze into each other's eyes and hold this position for three minutes. It works wonders!

## Kissing Hands (learning to love yourself)

I know this may sound a bit weird, but I'm sure by now you have noticed that Kundalini yoga has that element of being 'different', to say the least! There's always a lot of giggling when I do this one in workshops and classes, but I've also seen it bring tears to people's eyes. Leave your mind outside while you are doing this, otherwise you will not fully feel the benefits of it.

Lie down on your back with your hands by your side. Slowly bring your left hand to your mouth and kiss it, while visualizing receiving love. Then kiss your right hand and imagine giving love – to yourself, first. When you are comfortable with it, you can extend your thoughts to receiving and giving love to others.

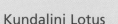

## Kundalini Lotus

This helps open up the sexual energy so that it can flow properly, and maintains potency. It can help if you're having problems letting go into orgasm, as can many of the positions for the second chakra (see page 76 in the chapter on Detox & De-stress).

Sit down in Easy Pose (see page 18) and take a firm hold on your big toes. Find a balance on your sitting bones, then open your legs wide and begin breathing evenly in and out of your nose in the Breath of Fire (see page 77). Close your eyes and try to relax. Hold for one to three minutes. This can be quite hard, and at first you might have difficulty finding your balance. If you cannot spread your legs wide at first, bend your knees.

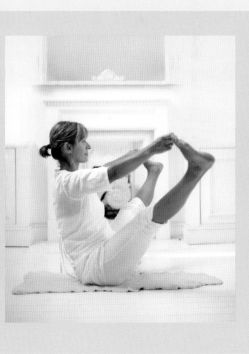

## Heart Energizer

An exercise to draw energy into the heart area and clear anxiety.

Sit in Easy Pose (see page 18). With straight elbows, extend your arms sixty degrees up and as far to the left as possible, keeping your upper body facing straight forward. Place the fingers of your right hand against the fingers of your left and lock the thumbs to hold the position. With eyes closed, inhale powerfully through the nose and exhale powerfully through the mouth until no more air is left in your navel. Carry on for up to five minutes.

To finish, inhale deeply, exhale completely, and hold for twenty seconds. Relax.

## Meditation for Inviting Love

This is for opening your heart to receive love: self-love, and the love of others. It also helps people who are in a relationship but find it's not gelling. I taught this to a class in Hong Kong a couple of years ago, and on a subsequent visit a student told me she had met someone in the lift afterwards. They hit it off between floors, exchanged numbers and married several months later!

Keeping your eyes closed, focus on the point between your eyebrows and repeat the mantra 'Sat Kar Tar'. Roll the 'r' each time, and keep the emphasis evenly on each syllable. As you say 'Sat', press your hands together in prayer pose. As you say 'Kar', extend your hands out from the shoulders halfway towards the final position. As you say 'Tar', fully extend your arms out to the sides, parallel to the floor.

Do this for three minutes, then relax your hands in Gyan Mudra (see page 19) and stay in meditation, allowing your body to settle. Build up until you can repeat the mantra for eleven minutes.

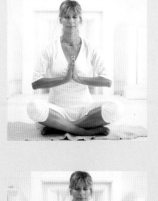

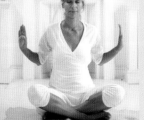

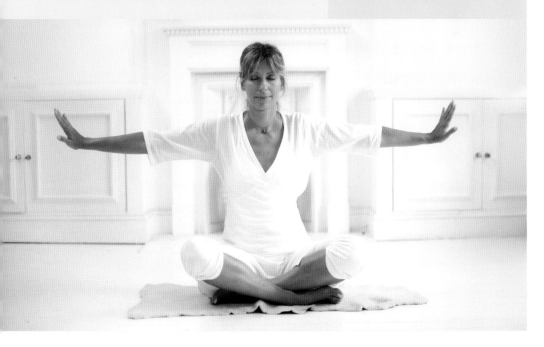

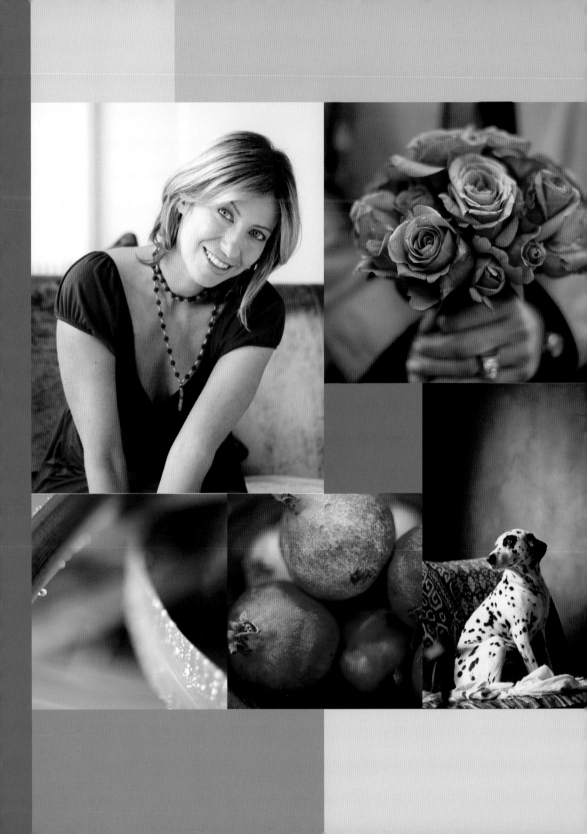

# Staying Youthful

# THROAT CHAKRA

THE FIFTH CHAKRA IS SITUATED IN THE THROAT, where the thyroid gland is found, so it is closely connected with your metabolism, how your hormones work. When it is blocked, people may experience throat complaints, voice problems, neck problems and thyroid imbalances.

We're now moving to the upper triangle, the last three chakras, which are more concerned with higher mental states and spirituality. This chakra is the last to be associated with an element, and the element here is ether – a subtle, heavenly energy, said to be from beyond Earth.

This energy centre is all about truth, about listening to that inner voice and discovering your authentic self. It's about the power of words, about language, knowledge, and the ability to communicate effectively – something we all need when dealing with children. When the throat chakra is open, we become very concerned with what we are saying. To put it bluntly: no more bullshit! If it is not working properly, you'll experience lethargy, weakness in your expressive or descriptive abilities, shyness, insecurity, fear of other people's opinions and judgements.

GOVERNS:
Truth

SHADOW
EMOTIONS:
Denial,
abruptness

COLOUR:
Blue

SYMBOL:
A lotus with
sixteen petals

ELEMENT:
Ether

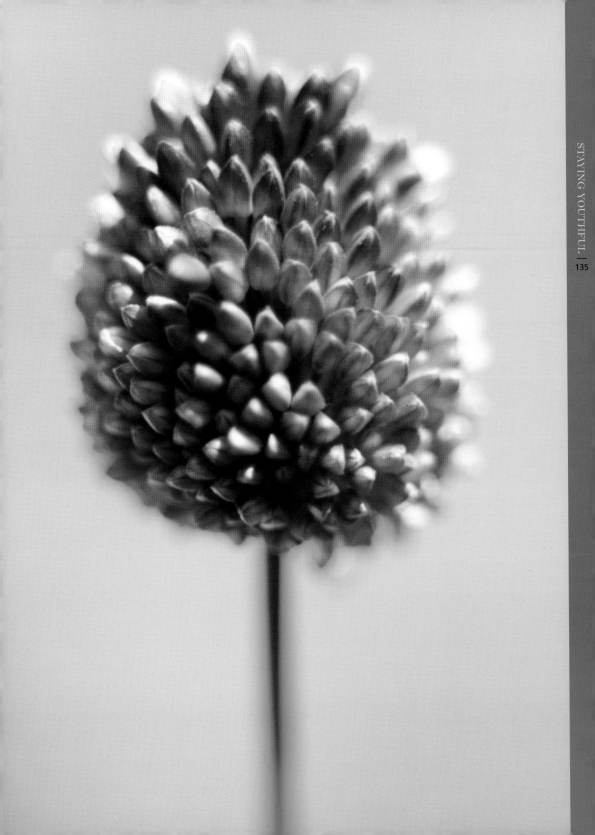

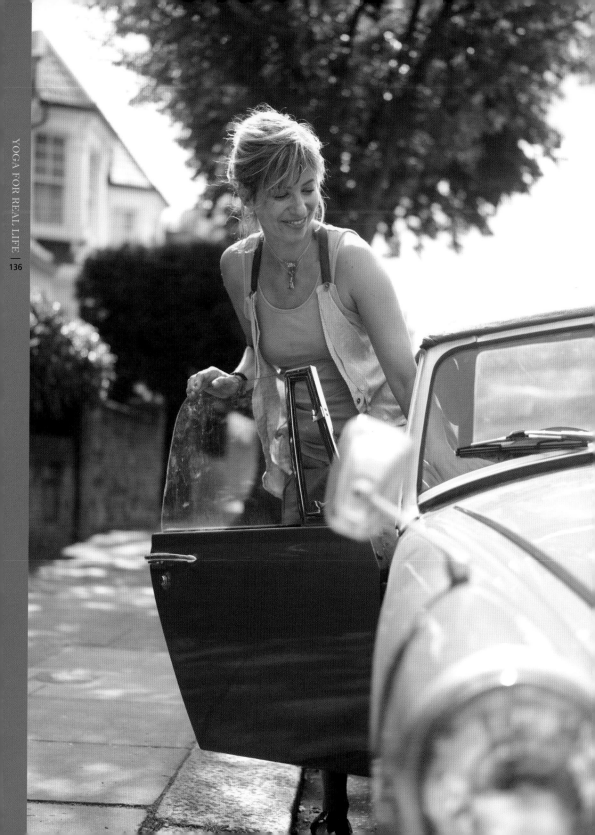

# Keep young and beautiful

AGEING IS SOMETHING THAT MANY OF US FEAR, but none of us can avoid. You are older now than when you started reading this paragraph! We can be so busy trying to hold back the years that we forget to celebrate how much we have learned, to be grateful for how far we have come. I for one wouldn't want to go back to the insecurity of my teenage years, or to the somewhat blinkered ambition of my twenties. And the aches and pains of later life are not inevitable. Nor are they totally irreversible.

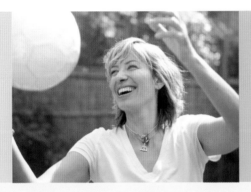

As you get older, you start getting rigid in the spine, which is our main column, our centre. If you don't do anything about it, the spinal fluid doesn't circulate and toxins get stuck there. From there it's all downhill, because you're not being rejuvenated, you're not juicing up the spine so you can just jump out of a chair instead of easing yourself up slowly. You can see how stiff people become. If you are flexible in the spine, you are flexible in the mind, you are open to new experiences. Increased circulation of the spinal fluid is linked to a good memory, something we lose as we get older.

Of course there's wear and tear on our bodies with age, but we speed it up with our stress and nervousness, by forgetting to breathe properly and by being so stiff that there isn't a good supply of blood and oxygen to the cells. A full hour of proper breath in a yoga session is better for you than anything you can imagine.

It's never too late to start. You're never too stiff to do this. You may not get into the full positions – at least not straight away – but that's not important. Start slowly. Listen to your body, be aware of how it feels. It's when you're not aware that you can get yourself too far into a position and end up in pain. Just do the warm-ups at first. Then try the Five Tibetans (see page 148) at the end of this chapter, all of which are designed to loosen up and strengthen the spine. If you're reading this and thinking, 'But I can't,' I'd say just try it for a few weeks and see how you feel. You'll have more energy, and you'll feel incredible – it will take years off you.

Even if you're young and doing lots of aerobic exercise, you need to spend time stretching your body and giving the joints space to relax after that workout. I've met lots of people who have found a new flexibility in later life through yoga. At my classes and retreats I've also met plenty (men especially) who are fit, muscular, they work out regularly and they look great. But they can't even touch their toes!

worse: her migraines had become so bad that she'd had brain scans and was on the waiting list to try out a new experimental drug.

The first time she tried Kundalini, she felt instantly energized. She started doing a little every day, and an hour-long session a couple of times a week, and her life was transformed.

'I put a lot of things down to middle age. My breathing wasn't the same. I used to get pains in my calves. My circulation wasn't good. Before I started doing this, we were going to spend £3,000 on a new bed, because I seriously thought there was something wrong with my back. It used to take me five minutes to get up in the

## 'I put a lot of things down to middle age... I used to get pains in my calves before I started doing this.'

Jacqui was in her forties when she discovered Kundalini yoga. She'd always been a size ten, but after her third son was born she couldn't wear many of her clothes: her tummy and waist were flabby, and parts of her body looked untoned. She joined a gym and began swimming twenty lengths every morning, went running regularly as well as walking three miles every day to take her son to and from nursery, and worked out with weights a couple of times a week. 'I hated every minute of it,' she admits. 'And after eighteen months, I really couldn't see any difference.' Her back started aching in the night and sometimes she struggled to get out of bed in the morning, and some long-term health problems were getting

morning! I put it down to the Caesarean, having a third child, being forty-three. But then suddenly I was jumping out of bed and I could do gymnastics I hadn't been able to do since I was eighteen. Now none of my clothes fit me any more, and I have to tumble-dry my jeans because I'm a size eight! My headaches have gone, and I've not taken medicine for months.

'It's become a little ritual for me, my yoga. I light my scented candle, shut the door and it's just me. It's very peaceful and relaxing. You're taking time for yourself, aren't you? My husband really encourages it, and although the kids make fun of me a bit, they know it's a good thing. They certainly don't dare disturb me when I'm doing it!'

'We don't stop playing
because we grow old;
we grow old because
we stop playing.'

GEORGE BERNARD SHAW
(1856–1950)

# Middle youth: a second lease of life

I WAS BORN IN 1963, which makes me one of the last of the baby boomers, the huge numbers of people who were born in the post-war years. There are a lot of us and we have money to spend, which is why Western culture has been so accommodating to us. When we began reaching our forties, for instance, some canny women's magazine rebranded this age as 'middle youth', because women in their forties and fifties just didn't act or feel middle-aged any more. It's very normal to want to start something new at this age. It's natural – you have more time to yourself, an opportunity to try new things, to learn and study new skills.

When I turned forty, I felt there was a change coming, that it was time for something new. When we decided to leave London and move to Santa Monica, to me it was important to leave almost everything behind. New house, new country, new furniture, new life by the ocean in California. It's been an exciting time for us, and it really feels like a fresh start, the opening of an entirely new chapter.

Looking back now, I see my earlier years as quite frustrating and painful at times. Like most of my friends, I was very insecure about my looks, about who I was. I'm so grateful I no longer have to deal with all that. We're given youth, and all the gorgeousness of it, but no confidence. As we get older we learn to accept the way we are, but we no longer have the youth. Still, I'd rather be here, now, than be young and self-conscious again. Confidence is a beautiful place to be in, and it only comes from wisdom, age and experience.

I've got to the point where I feel I'm starting fresh all over again, and it's so exciting. I feel I'm finding out who I am, so I can do things in a different way – different thoughts, different mind. For me, this is the best part. This is our time to soar, it's harvest time. You've gone through those anxiety-filled years of youth, and now you have perspective, and you know what's important in your life, what your priorities are.

Before, you're busy achieving, then you're occupied with your family, often juggling children and work. Then that starts to take care of itself, and it's your time. It's an opportunity to reinvent yourself, to no longer feel trapped by any wrong choices you may have made earlier. So as we make this transition from the first part of life to the next, it's important to analyse our patterns, habits and behaviour and allow ourselves to be open-minded, making way for new experiences. Challenging how you did things in the past is a great way to improve your future. Try things you haven't done before, and use yoga and

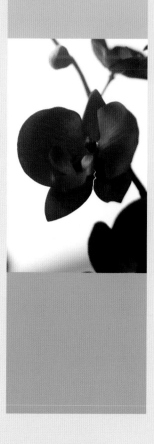

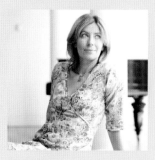

meditation to ask yourself what it is you *really* want now. And remember, you've earned the right to have all the pleasure your body can experience! You've already been the good mother, the caring housewife, and built a career. From this point on, any new accomplishments should be things you do for yourself, not for outside approval.

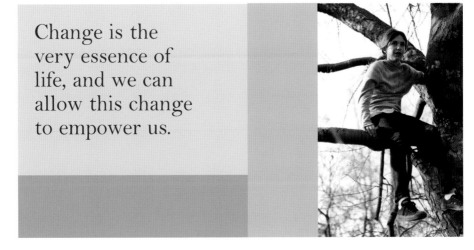

Change is the very essence of life, and we can allow this change to empower us.

With menopause, women are given a very physical reminder that a new phase of life is beginning. Our biology is closely linked to nature's cycles – the waxing and waning of the moon, the ebb and flow of the tides, the changes of the seasons – and these are reflected in the female menstrual cycle. At the mid-point of our period, for example, when we are ovulating, we are more receptive to others and to new ideas – more 'fertile'. We often feel sexier at this time, and our bodies secrete hormones that reflect this. After ovulation, as the moon wanes, we become more reflective and inward. Just as our intuition varies during the different phases of our menstrual period, it changes again after we go through

menopause – when we no longer menstruate. This can be a time of great change and new possibilities for a woman. We are open to new creative energies and profound transformation. Change is the very essence of life, and we can allow this change to empower us.

The exercises for adrenals on page 76 are very important at this time, as are the pelvic floor exercises on page 176. The key to navigating the waves of change in our sexual cycle is to learn to do so willingly – to go with the flow from puberty through the child-bearing years to menopause. Trust your ability to transform, and appreciate the particular qualities and rewards in each different stage on our journey.

# Ageing gracefully – and gratefully

Every time you think it's too late to start something new, remind yourself that Pablo Picasso continued to make innovative art right up to his death at the age of ninety-one. Barbara Castle, the Labour minister who broke new ground for women in British politics, was still active in the House of Lords right up to her death in 2002, aged ninety-one. When the novelist Doris Lessing accepted the Nobel Prize for Literature in 2007 with a fiery speech on global inequality, she was eighty-seven. Popular music is full of icons now old enough to qualify for a free bus pass, from Tina Turner to the Rolling Stones, while classical musicians and conductors seem to go on for ever.

Make a promise to your body that you will take good care of it. Stay in shape, live a healthy lifestyle and don't ever use lines like 'I am too old for that.' Instead, your mantra should be 'I am wise, capable and I can do anything.'

Something I learned from Deepak Chopra is to repeat an affirmation every day, setting your mental age fifteen years younger than your biological one. Throughout the day, whenever you see your reflection, greet yourself and say to yourself, 'I am a radiant healthy woman.' Visualize yourself as that woman, and see yourself standing erect with good posture. Take time to give gratitude to every moment of your life, to everything you already have.

> Don't ever use lines like 'I am too old for that.' Instead, your mantra should be 'I am wise, capable and I can do anything.

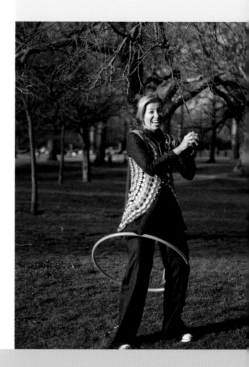

## Beautiful inside *and* out

In many societies the old are revered for their wisdom and experience, but our society tends to worship youth, and the older you are, the more invisible you might feel. Many women spend their middle years desperately buying every lotion and potion and even undergoing surgery to try and hold on to that youth, but to me it's so beautiful to see a woman with the lines of wisdom on her face, especially when she also looks healthy, smiling and content. Of course she has lines – she's lived a great life! If you mature with nothing showing on your face, what a boring life you must have led. Every one of those lines tells a story, and if your man can't accept you and your life story, he's the wrong man.

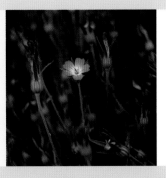

## You're never too old

It's always interesting looking at the faces in my classes during meditation. The years just melt away from people. Some of them look like children again! If you're after an instant anti-ageing formula, I can't think of a better one. Yoga in general makes you feel more confident, reminds you just how wonderful you already are. You learn to accept yourself, and then everyone will accept you too.

I recently met a lady at an all-day workshop who had taken up yoga at the age of seventy-four, after her husband died. A decade later, she had a network of friends all over the world that she'd met on yoga holidays, she was full of laughter and life, and she was more flexible than many people half her age. So remember, you're never too old. Just do it. Go and do all the wild things you ever dreamed of doing, all the things you never learned and wanted to. All the things you were to scared to do, all the places you wanted to see – now is the time! It's never too late.

## THE HEALING POWER OF LAUGHTER

I RECENTLY DISCOVERED LAUGHTER YOGA. It is – ahem! – 'laughably' simple, yet it absolutely hits the spot as a mini-yoga workout. The brainchild of Dr Madan Kataria, it has become incredibly successful, and there are now over 6,000 laughter groups in more than sixty countries worldwide.

Dr Kataria began by instructing a group of us to simply simulate laughter. It is very infectious, and soon everyone was laughing for real. After a few minutes I was surprised how exhausted I was, but we all felt an incredible high. It seems the maxim 'laughter is the best medicine' is true. When you laugh, you breathe in a way you never do otherwise, even in a yoga class, releasing all those nerves in the face. It stimulates the immune system to release endorphins, the body's natural painkiller, giving a feeling of well-being while reducing stress, depression and anxiety. Laughter also helps to control blood pressure by reducing the release of stress-related hormones; it increases our oxygen supply, alleviates pain, ensures good sleep and reduces snoring because it is very good for the muscles of the soft palate and throat. All that and it's fun, too!

The incredible thing is that the body doesn't need to know if the laughter is real or simulated to trigger a positive effect.

So try it! Burst out into laughter, and carry on until your stomach hurts. Nothing can beat a good belly laugh. You'll feel full of fire and life.

'The most wasted of all days is one without laughter.'

E E CUMMINGS (1894–1962)

# TIPS

## HERBAL SUPPLEMENTS FOR MIDDLE YOUTH

AS YOU APPROACH MENOPAUSE and during this important transition time, take red clover extract – available in tablet form online or from health food stores – three times a day to help with hot flushes and night sweats and generally re-balance the hormones naturally.

Also try liquid herbal extracts: put twenty drops of stinging nettle, twenty drops of sage per day into a glass of water.

And take lots of evening primrose oil! Capsules are sold at most good health shops.

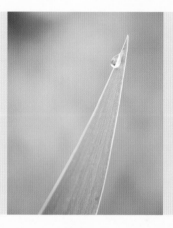

## FACIAL MASSAGE TO REDUCE WRINKLES

Massage the neck from top to bottom lightly with your fingers. All your glands are here, and if you feel a cold coming on, massaging your throat and neck is great. Drain the glands, moving up and down in a circular movement with both hands. Really go under the chin. Then go over the same area, moving to left and right.

Now move from your temples down along the jaw in a circular motion. Using your index fingers, make overlapping half-circles across your forehead, kneading the skin from side to side, then up and down.

Squeeze the skin at the outer edge of your eyebrows, furthest from the nose.

Then lightly tap around the eye socket – along the line of your eyebrows and under your eyes, just tapping away all the puffiness and increasing circulation.

Press your fingertips down on either side of your nose about a centimetre up from the nostril – it should be almost painful if you're pressing the right spot, clearing the sinuses.

Finally, put your hands in prayer position with your nose between them, and sweep your fingertips firmly up the cheekbones on each side. Finish by tapping your cheeks, forehead and neck.

# TIPS

## DEALING WITH ACHES AND PAINS

THE WARM-UP EXERCISES at the start of this book are easy, enjoyable, and work wonders for everyday aches and pains. Rolling your wrists and ankles in a clockwise, then anti-clockwise direction also helps flexibility, especially when you've been sitting for long periods.

When I get twinges, I close my eyes, and I just say in my head, 'Love. Knowingness. Bliss.' And wherever the pain is, I send a pulsing light to it. I visualize it, and keep sending white light and love. It's amazing how effective it is, and how quickly it works!

## THE POWER OF VISUALIZATION

THIS FIFTH CHAKRA is also closely connected with visualization. Here are two ways you might want to play with this skill.

### MOOD BOARDS
At the start of every year or the beginning of a new project, I make mood boards of everything I want to achieve. I cut out images and headlines from magazines to illustrate what I wish to bring into being. These can range from lifestyle treats, say an infinity pool in a luxurious island resort, to family pictures showing your children looking happy, healthy and glowing. You might want to add a photo of relatives whose good health you pray for, even the balance you'd like to see in your bank account. Essentially, anything you can invest positive thought into. Put the board somewhere you will glimpse it often. You have sent the message out, so let go of it. No more 'I wish', just 'What I project out I will receive back.'

### ASKING FOR INSPIRATION
Sometimes, however hard we try, the ideas just don't come. There's a lot of truth in the old adage, 'Sleep on it.' Our subconscious mind will continue to process the problem unhindered in dream state and the solution will present itself when we wake. Here's a more poetic way of doing it. Before you go to bed, visualize writing a message detailing your problem or concern on beautiful manuscript paper. Tie the paper with an imaginary red ribbon, put it into an ornate box and write the name of the recipient on the box. This could be an angel, divine power or departed loved one, even a friend, relative or lover who may have a solution. Now imagine tying a balloon to the box. Let the box go and watch it float up into the night sky. Bless it on its journey, because a reply will be sent to you in the morning. It's as if sharing the problem with an imaginary other removes the burden we put on ourselves to find a solution. Once free of this, the answer appears.

# RECIPE

## Talk to Me

This shake is excellent for the thyroid and
metabolic process. Coconut water cleans
and heals the thyroid and parathyroid
glands. Kids love this, and it could help
them hear what adults are trying to tell
them.

240–480ml (1–2 cups) coconut water
    (see page 68), or coconut juice
    (you could also add raw fresh coconut)
good handful of blueberries
1 tablespoon almonds
1 date, pitted and chopped
    into small pieces
good squeeze of lemon juice
raw honey to taste
pinch of ground cinnamon

Place everything in a blender
and purée until smooth and
creamy. Serve with a loud,
spoken 'Thank you!'

# EXERCISES

## The First Tibetan

This works on your inner ear, and your balance. It's great for fighting ageing.

Stand up straight, with your arms outstretched to the sides. Fingers are together, palms open and facing downward. Holding this arm position, spin a full circle in a clockwise direction (if you turn your head to the right, that is the direction in which you want to spin). Repeat. At the beginning try just a few spins, and see how you feel. Keep adding more, until you can spin twenty-one times without a break. You may experience some dizziness when you first practise this exercise. Be careful, don't push it. With regular practice the dizziness will stop, and the spin will become easy and fluid, even at very fast speeds.

When you stop spinning, stand with your feet hip width apart and your hands on your hips. Take three full, deep breaths, inhaling through the nose and exhaling through the mouth. And relax.

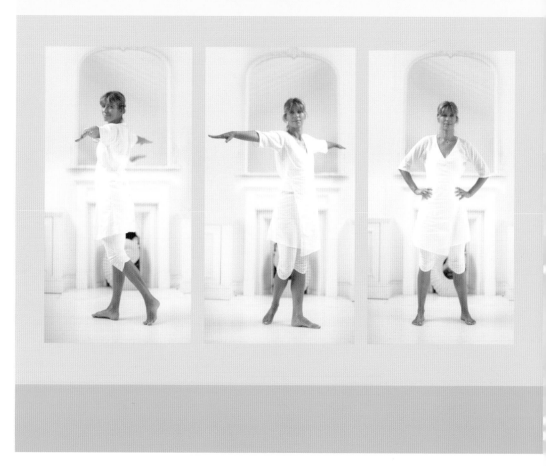

## The Second Tibetan

This strengthens the abdominal muscles and massages the organs. It also strengthens the digestive system and lower back.

Lie on your back on a mat or rug with your legs fully extended, toes pointed and touching. Put your arms by your sides, palms flat on the floor, or under your buttocks if you have a weak lower back. Inhale through your nose, lift your legs up as far as you can, toes pointing towards the ceiling, and lift your head and arms, tucking your chin into your chest. Exhale through either your nose or your mouth, bringing your legs and head down to the starting position, completely flat on the ground.

Build up until you are able to repeat the entire motion twenty-one times, inhaling as you raise your legs and head, exhaling as you bring them down.

When you are finished, stand with your feet hip width apart and your hands on your hips (see First Tibetan). Take three full, deep breaths, inhaling through the nose and exhaling through the mouth. And relax.

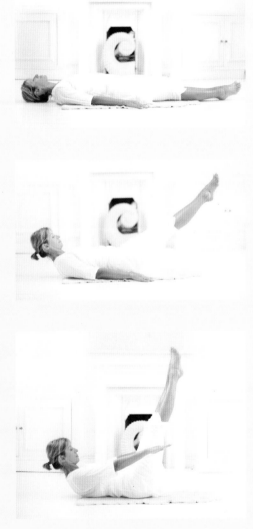

### The Third Tibetan

This is beneficial for the digestive and reproductive systems. It stretches the stomach and intestines, alleviating constipation. The backward bend loosens the vertebrae and stimulates the spinal nerves, relieving backache, lumbago, rounded back and drooping shoulders. By stretching the front of the neck you also tone the organs in this region and regulate the thyroid gland.

Kneel with the tops of your feet flat to the ground, heels in the air. Your knees should be about four inches apart. Place your palms against the backs of your thighs, just below the buttocks. Keep your spine straight, with your chin tucked into your chest. Inhale through the nose, arching back from the waist. Lift and open the chest. Drop your head as far back as you comfortably can. Your hands will support you as you lean back. Exhale through either your nose or your mouth as you return to the starting position. Build up until you can repeat the entire motion twenty-one times in a steady, unbroken rhythm.

When you finish, stand with your feet hip width apart and your hands on your hips (see First Tibetan). Take three full, deep breaths, inhaling through the nose and exhaling through the mouth. And relax.

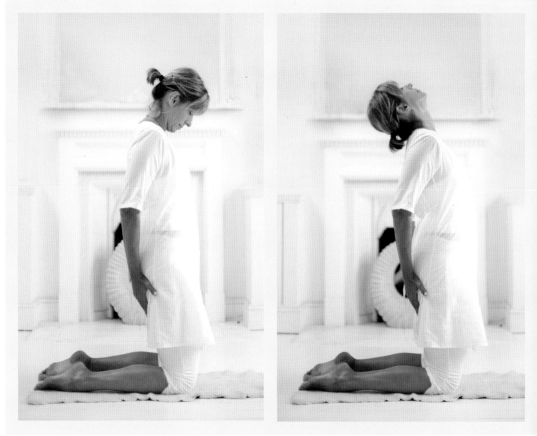

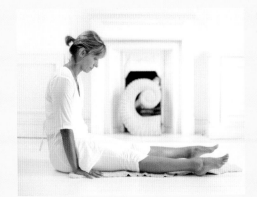

## The Fourth Tibetan

This tones the spine and is good for the nervous, digestive, respiratory, cardiovascular and glandular systems. In women, it influences hormonal secretions and helps to relieve a variety of gynaecological disorders.

Sit up straight on the floor, with your legs stretched out in front of you. Place the palms of your hands flat on the floor beside your hips. The position of the hands is very important: they must be placed exactly alongside the hips. Tuck your chin into your chest. Inhaling through your nose, raise your hips as you bend your knees, bringing the soles of your feet flat to the floor and dropping your head all the way back. Exhale through the nose as you come down to the starting position. Build up until you can repeat this motion twenty-one times in a steady, unbroken rhythm.

Finish by standing with your feet hip width apart and your hands on your hips (see First Tibetan). Take three full, deep breaths, inhaling through the nose and exhaling through the mouth. And relax.

### The Fifth Tibetan

This posture relieves backache and keeps the spine supple and healthy. A stiff spine interferes with the nervous impulses from the brain to the body and vice versa, so arching the spine improves circulation in the back region and tones the nerves.

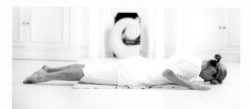

Lie on your stomach, with your palms flat on the floor beside your shoulders. Both the arms and the legs should be about two feet apart. Push your upper body up with your arms, tilting your head up and back. This is called Cobra Pose. Keep your arms and legs straight, inhaling through your nose as you raise your buttocks and tuck your chin into your chest, bringing your body up into a perfect triangle. Exhale through your nose as you swing back down to the starting position. Your arms and legs should not bend at all. Build up until you can repeat the entire motion twenty-one times in a smooth, unbroken rhythm.

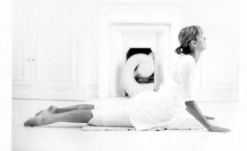

If you find this too difficult, you can also work the spine by moving from Cow to Cat Pose. Kneel on all fours, knees directly under your hips, hands level with your shoulders, index fingers pointing forwards. Use a mat, folded blanket or cushions if this makes your knees sore. As you inhale, curve your spine down towards the floor, and put your head back, looking towards the sky. As you exhale, arch your spine upwards and let your head hang down in a relaxed way, looking towards your navel.

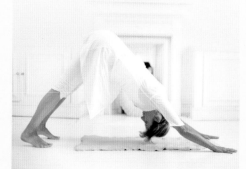

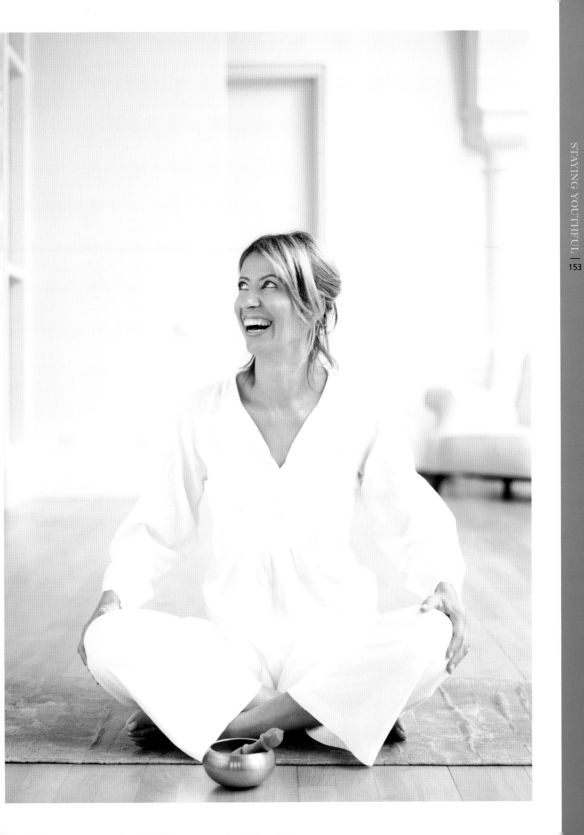

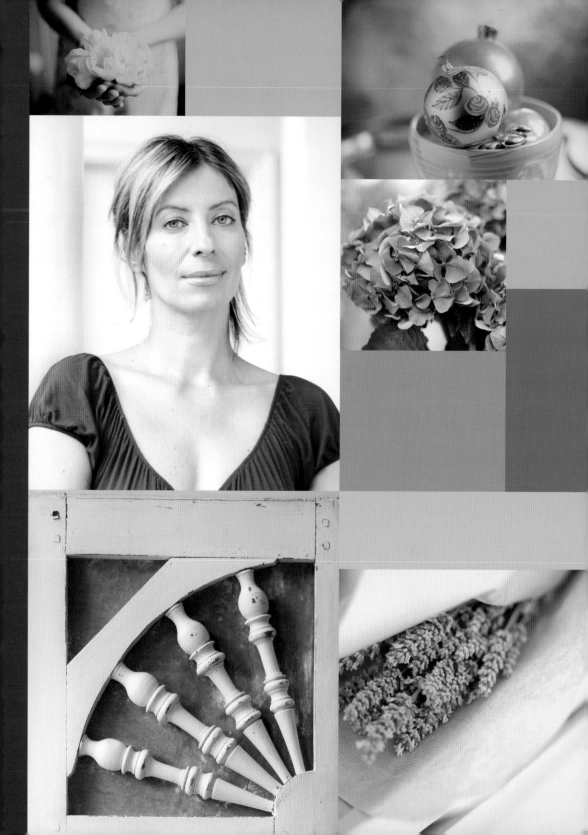

# Children

# THIRD EYE CHAKRA

THE SIXTH CHAKRA IS RIGHT BETWEEN YOUR EYEBROWS, the place we often focus on when closing our eyes for meditation. It's the third eye, the eye that sees inwards. Physically, it is connected with the pituitary gland, which releases serotonin – the neurotransmitter most responsible for our mood (people with depression tend to have low serotonin levels).

Working on this energy centre opens up our vision, our intuition. When it is blocked, you have no faith in anything, no connection to a greater whole. You tend to live for material things, for money, not being aware or conscious or sharing. You see only what you experience with your senses, rather than going deeper.

| GOVERNS: | SHADOW EMOTIONS: | COLOUR: | SYMBOL: | ELEMENT: |
|---|---|---|---|---|
| Intuition | Confusion, depression | Indigo | A lotus with two petals | None |

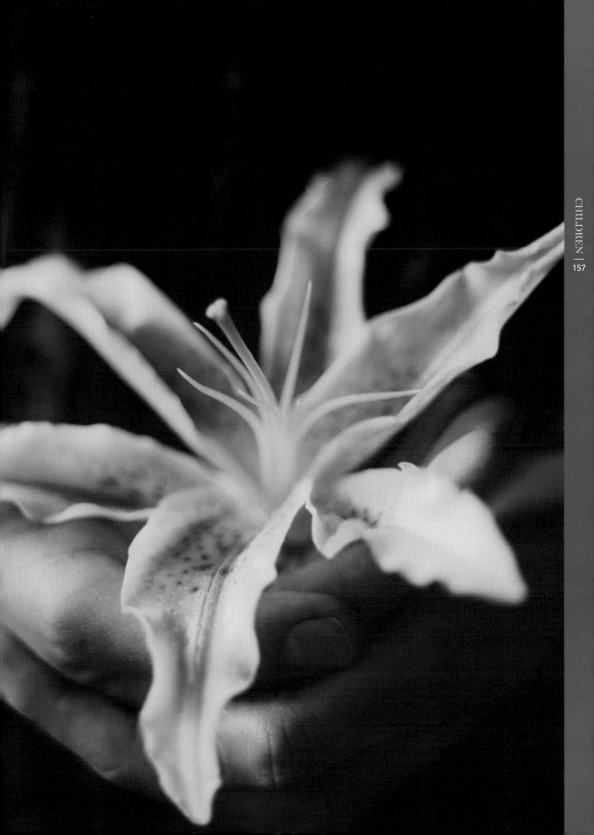

# Pregnancy and birth

'The purest thing in the world is the heart of the mother. It can move the Universe.'

YOGI BHAJAN (1929–2004)

THERE COMES A TIME FOR MOST WOMEN when they know their hearts are mother-ready. Some say it's the biological clock ticking, but the beating of the heart and its readiness to share love is equally important. When I reached thirty-three, I knew with absolute certainty that I was ready to begin the journey into motherhood.

## Getting married and letting go

Magnus and I married in December 1995. The wedding was a fairytale, candlelit winter-evening affair. It meant a lot to me that my greatest friends were there, but having my mother by my side meant the most. She was battling terminal cancer, an illness she had ignored until it was all but too late, yet somehow she kept going despite her frailty and weakness. She was determined to share this moment with me.

Sadly but inevitably, the wedding was followed only weeks later by my mother's funeral, which was solemn, grey and simple – in every way the opposite of the joyful celebration a few weeks earlier. We cremated her, and would later return her ashes to Macedonia and bury them next to my father's. Apart from my brother, Dejan, I had no family left to speak of, so my desire to have children burned stronger.

## Conceiving

A few months later, to my amazement, I took a pregnancy test and I tested positive. Magnus used to tell me how his mother knew the exact moment each of her six children was conceived, but I never felt I could be so certain. However, what was beyond all doubt was that I was to be a mother.

For those who are not finding it so easy to conceive, Kundalini can help enormously: Bridge Pose (see page 77) is particularly useful. There are many studies suggesting that regular yoga and meditation can help with infertility. It's also true that there are few things in life more stressful than being unable to conceive a baby when you desperately want one, and the exercises in this book can at the very least help with the resulting stress and anxiety.

## Being pregant and giving birth

I loved being pregnant. I was incredibly lucky: I never had morning sickness, I felt physically and emotionally amazing and my skin glowed. I never felt heavy or put on much weight, apart from the small but perfect bump in my belly. I grew in confidence and loved showing off my sleek roundness. I even did some modelling work where I proudly displayed my pregnant tummy.

Cheyenne was born in December 1996, a year after our wedding. Yoga can be an excellent way to prepare for birth, which is why there are now so many classes for expectant mothers around the country. But no matter how prepared you are, nature may have her own ideas.

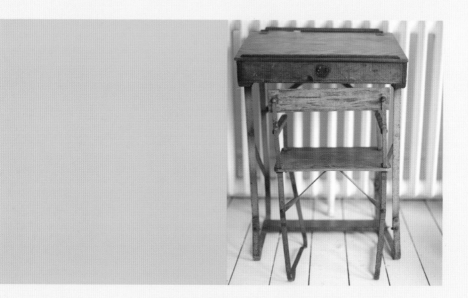

In my case, the birth proved long-winded, painful and difficult. I had planned a natural delivery, but I was in labour for three days and reached exhaustion point. After thirty-six hours I agreed to an epidural. It may be unfashionable to say so, but I'm not sure if I could have managed without it. So much for the 'keep it natural' promise I had made myself! The final contractions were really tough, but the moment Cheyenne appeared, all that pent-up love and expectation gave way to tears of joy.

I believe the struggle to bring a child into the world creates an important bond. We have journeyed so far together and are forever bound through this act of creativity. We are cocoon and butterfly.

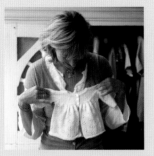

Yoga can be an excellent way to prepare for birth, which is why there are now so many classes for expectant mothers.

## Alone with your baby

Home from hospital, the scary truth dawned: how on earth do I do this? How do I hold her? She keeps crying: is she in pain, is something wrong? Do I call a doctor? On the one hand we have this strong instinct to create life, but many of us barely hold a baby until we take our own home. We can feel completely helpless when it comes to coping with this tiny, vulnerable, cooing and pooing creature.

Suddenly I doubted my abilities as a mum, and while most of us have mothers or mothers-in-law queuing up to offer help and advice, needed or not, I had neither, and felt quite alone. Luckily help was on hand in the shape of Razia, a Kosovan refugee who was also a brilliant and highly trained maternity nurse. She took matters in hand with a no-nonsense but loving efficiency, guiding me through everything from nappy rash and colic to Albanian lullabies that could put an insomniac wrestler to sleep. Razia's help would prove invaluable during those difficult and exhausting first few months, and again when my second daughter was born. She restored my confidence in my mothering abilities.

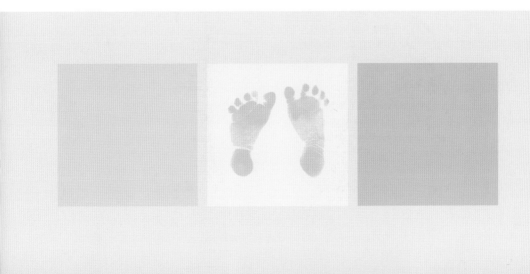

### Breastfeeding

The next challenge was feeding. I wanted more than anything to breastfeed – I saw it as another important bonding ritual between mother and child, and I also believe strongly in the superior nutritional value of breast milk. After the first few feeds, however, my nipples became red and swollen and agonizingly sensitive. Each feed would leave me in tears, mainly of disappointment. I tried expressing milk, but at this point I learned that I had developed chronic mastitis. Reluctantly, after trying all kinds of alternative remedies, I took the antibiotics the doctor offered me and gave up breastfeeding.

### Coping with more than one...

Two years later, my second daughter, Shanti was born. While looking after one baby was exhilarating and full of novel experiences, two was more of a challenge. I remember feeling permanently grumpy and miserable from lack of sleep. I felt I couldn't cope, and once again the doubts set in. I found it harder to bond with Shanti, and developed what was eventually diagnosed as post-natal depression. Once it was explained that my feelings were a direct result of hormonal imbalances brought on by the birth and not some deep-seated case of self-loathing and baby allergy, I knew I could do something about it. I had not practised yoga for weeks before the birth, and had lost the will during my depression, but now I began putting simple yoga sets together. After a few days the dark clouds lifted, and when I held Shanti I was filled with love and happiness.

I developed post-natal depression... I began putting simple yoga sets together. After a few days the dark clouds lifted.

## Watching them grow

Watching characters develop is endlessly fascinating. Each day brings a new miracle. The rewards so outweighed the difficult moments. By the time the girls were a few years old, however, it was clear to me that I did not want any more children. Perhaps it was because I was one of only two siblings myself and didn't have the personal experience of a big, bustling family to draw on. Whatever the reasons, I think we have to listen to our bodies and hearts rather than external pressures and expectations. Women now have more control over their fertility than ever before, and the choice should always be ours.

I recently met an amazing family with eight children between the ages of two and twenty-two. Their mother, Clarissa, glowed with beauty and vitality, and presided over them all with an effortless air of serenity. All the children were incredibly well balanced and charming. Magnus's mother, Jini, had six children under the age of seven at one stage, and although their family life was fairly chaotic and times were hard, he and all his siblings tell of an idyllic childhood. Perhaps the more children you have the easier it becomes. What is clear, however, is that these women have mothering superpowers I could only dream of!

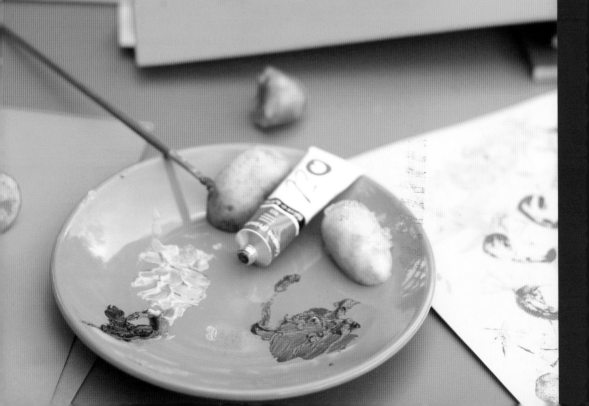

# Becoming your mother

ONE THING ABOUT MOTHERHOOD that no one warns you about is that we seem destined to become faithful replicas of our own mothers – and I'm not just talking about cake-baking!

## 'You may house their bodies but not their souls,
## For their souls dwell in the house of tomorrow'...

When I was growing up, my mother was very over-protective. Like many matriarchs she was determined, ambitious and self-righteous, and we soon learned to play by her rules or suffer the consequences. When I was a teenager she would insist I was home every evening at 10 p.m. I was terrified of overstepping the curfew, and I remember to this day the silhouette of her figure on the balcony of our apartment as she watched the road, waiting to interrogate me as to where I had been and with whom. I became so embarrassed by her that I dared not bring friends back (and forget boyfriends!). None of my friends was ever good or trustworthy enough for her, and any pursuit I engaged in apart from the piano she considered unladylike or too dangerous.

## ...'You may strive to be like them,
## but seek not to make them like you'...

Although I was happily aware that I had inherited my mother's drive and ambition, I was shocked when Magnus began to point out how overbearing and over-protective I could be with Cheyenne and Shanti. I would barely let them go to the corner shop, even when Cheyenne was eleven. Recently, when Magnus wanted to take them flying in a small plane, I did everything I could to persuade him against it. When he told me he had taken them rock-climbing and proudly showed me pictures of them scrambling up a precipitous mountainside, it took everything I had to stifle a scream.

## ...'For life goes not backward nor tarries with yesterday'...

We learn so much that is useful from our parents. As children we assume they are wise and perfect, and it's not until we are grown up ourselves, and have to deal with the same issues and dilemmas of parenthood, that we begin to understand our parents and love them for who they are: real people with flaws and imperfections, strengths and weaknesses and issues of their own – some, no doubt, inherited from their parents before them. In my case not all my memories were idyllic, so it was important for me to make peace with my mother and no longer harbour resentment about the past.

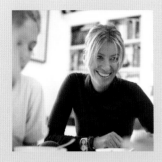

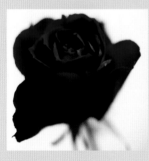

...'You are the bows from which your children as living arrows are sent forth.'

So my mothering mantra is 'Let go, and find balance.' Our children are like birds that will fly the nest all too soon, and we mustn't clip their wings or hold them back when nature says it is their time to soar. We must refrain from being the interfering matriarch who refuses to acknowledge that her child is a fully formed individual and no longer a baby. The greatest test of how well we've brought our kids up is how much common sense and initiative they have. If we can help them develop a strong moral compass, then teach them to read the danger signs when they are out on their own and understand empathetically the minds of others, they will be truly ready to take on the world.

(Quote from *The Prophet* by Kahlil Gibran)

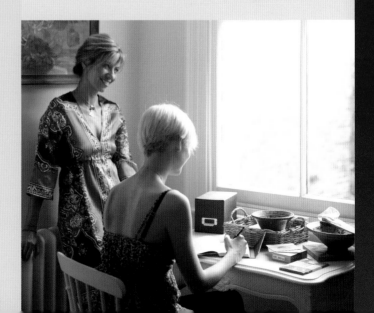

# That elusive work/life balance

ONE OF THE FIRST of my close friends to give birth was Pauline, an avid windsurfer and extreme sports wonderwoman. Shortly after the birth we drove down to West Wittering in West Sussex, where she and her partner were making the most of a perfect windy day to sail. Pauline had little India strapped to her in a front harness and was going about her business completely unhindered. It's true that children needn't stop us doing anything we want to do, but being a mother can be a career in itself.

Whatever we choose to do, there is always a degree of guilt involved. Parents obsess about giving their children 'quality time', but all too often this means trying too hard, buying unnecessary things, scheduling trips and fun activities, when what they really want is time with you.

In my life, my children come first. But I don't fuss unnecessarily, or make myself continuously available as their live-in personal assistant/maid/taxi driver. Try to prioritize what is really important: love, shelter, support, and an environment that cultivates free-thinking, enquiring minds.

## Snap! The job's a game!

Make time for them by including them in chores, for instance. Sorting the laundry with a toddler can be fun if you're not in too much of a hurry, while dusting or mopping can turn into a great game if you lose your perfectionist streak. When they're very young, making dinner with them can be excruciatingly slow, but can provide the connection you yearn for. Boys in particular are far more likely to open up and start talking to you if you're engaged in a task together, and patience in the early years can pay dividends. I have a friend whose twelve-year-old now makes dinner for the family, on his own, a couple of nights a week. He gets a huge confidence boost from his growing culinary skills, and from feeling he has contributed, and his meals have become relaxed, festive family events.

Children can teach us a lot about time. No one has told them there is a shortage of it in the modern world.

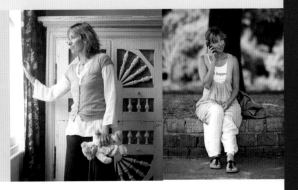

## Let them teach you, too

Anyone who has tried to get a toddler out of the door in a hurry can testify that a child can teach you all you need to know about patience and temper control. Somehow the more you hurry them, the slower they will go. But children can also teach us a lot about time. No one has told them there is a shortage of it in the modern world, so they take all the time they need to put on their shoes, make a finger painting, stare at a ladybird on a leaf. Let go and enjoy this moment with them, and you've given them something far more important than a new toy or designer outfit. Let them guide you, and you'll rediscover the fun of splashing in puddles, rolling down a grassy bank in summer, lying on a blanket just watching birds and clouds. And when time is really short, it's the little things that really matter: taking those few minutes to ask about their day and really listening when they answer; taking a second, when you sit down to eat, to make eye contact with everyone around the table and smile at them.

## Watching them grow

I want my girls to enjoy a more rounded and carefree childhood and discover their own potential at their own rate. We provide them with opportunities and when they find something they enjoy, such as a sport, or playing an instrument, we try to motivate them and encourage them.

Parents can exhaust themselves and their children by scheduling every day with activities, with no space to breathe. Left to find their own entertainment, kids will eventually start making things, inventing new games – they'll pick up a book or start using their imaginations. Or perhaps they'll just rest or daydream: both useful skills!

When I do mantra or meditate, I ask the Universe to guide me in letting go as a parent, and to help me accept that what will be will be. I ask for guidance in balancing discipline and freedom through the lens of unconditional love, that I may instil good qualities and virtues in my children yet allow them to flourish as themselves. I am eternally thankful for the incredible gift of motherhood.

# Teaching your child yoga

'Mama exhorted her children at every opportunity to "jump at de sun". We might not land on the sun, but at least we would get off the ground.' ZORA NEALE HURSTON (1891–1960)

SOME CHILDREN LOVE YOGA. At a recent mind and body festival I met Claire, a yoga teacher from Watford, and her six-year-old daughter, Hazel. Hazel had started watching my slots on the satellite TV channel Body in Balance, and doing the exercises with me.

'Both my daughters have been brought up with yoga,' Claire explained. 'From an early age, if I had my yoga mat out Hazel would just curl up on the end of it and watch me. She'd occasionally do yoga with me, but I've always felt it's best to be led by the children on things like that. I've taught yoga to teenagers, for instance, and the ones who stick with it are the ones who really want to do it, not those who've just come along with friends from school.

'Hazel started watching your show – she called you "Kundalini lady", and doing the movements with you. I record them all when she's at school, and it's become a ritual for her. Normally she's quite flighty, into anything and everything all at once, but when she's doing her Kundalini she's completely focused, to the exclusion of everything around her. Which is extraordinary, because she's never shown that focus with anything else!'

I also met a twelve-year-old who was a karate black belt, but had bonded with her six-year-old brother by doing yoga with him. But what really moves me is the letters from mothers saying that doing yoga together has bought them closer to their teenage daughters. Sometimes, when children hit their teens and start developing interests of their own, you grow apart, and yoga can be your thing, your time together.

I remember one very powerful letter in particular. This mother said her teenage daughter had been very rebellious and resentful, but since they'd been practising Kundalini together they'd regained their old closeness. The daughter had more focus in school, she was calmer and happier and was making much better choices when it came to friends.

It's widely accepted that doing yoga in pregnancy can make natural childbirth easier, but there are also growing numbers of classes where new mums can practise yoga with their babies, and children-only classes like Yogabugs are spreading nationwide too. Some kids really take to it, but it's best not to force it. And sometimes it's nice to be able to shut the door and do our yoga alone!

There are useful skills you can teach even very young children, like taking a deep breath to calm themselves, and kids love the shouting and chopping movements of the anger release exercise on page 106. The lymphatic drainage exercise on page 105 is great for kids too.

I was once invited to teach in a school for a few days. The students ranged from nine to seventeen, and every forty-five minutes I had a different age group. With one group, the other teachers said, 'Oh, this is the naughty class! Don't feel bad if you can't get them calm.'

At first they were all laughing but as soon as I gave them the lymphatic drainage position to do, they really got into it. It works on the whole body, and I'd keep them going at it for five or six minutes, which is hard. But being kids, and competitive, they were really responsive when I'd shout, 'You can do it! Work at it! Believe it!' They were so determined to make it, and they all kept going: nobody put their hands down. They loved it! Afterwards, you've cleared all the stagnated energies, the lymphatic system is all buzzed up and clearing, and you feel this huge rush of energy. When you stop, you really feel it. Straight away, I went into meditation, and all of them closed their eyes without a word. The other teachers couldn't believe it. They realized the benefits of introducing yoga into the school, especially before exams. It helped the kids sit down calmly with a clear head, and their grades improved as a result.

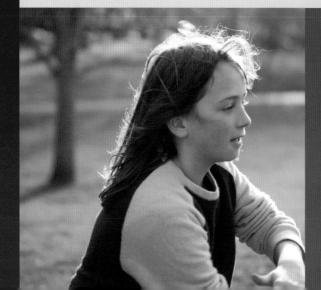

# Reaching out past the family

'We make a living by what we get, but we make a life by what we give.' WINSTON CHURCHILL (1874–1965)

At the heart of Yogi Bhajan's teaching is the importance of giving back to our fellow humans. This can begin at home with our children – they don't care as much about fancy toys as they do about having our time and attention. We get so caught up in the 'busy-ness' of life that sometimes we forget to set time aside for them. Reading together is a classic way of bonding, but so is telling them about your day, finding out about theirs, driving to and from soccer practice and giving up every Saturday morning to watch the game – the opportunities for self-sacrifice with our children are endless!

If we don't have children of our own, there are plenty of under-privileged kids who can benefit from a little of our time. After-school programmes are often in great need of adults to help children with their homework: I have a friend who shares her love of art by donating her time to teach a weekly art class at a school whose budget cannot afford such a 'luxury'. She says she gets as much pleasure from it as the kids do. Or we can 'adopt' or sponsor a child through a charity like Save the Children. The ways to give back to the world are varied and numerous – volunteer programmes are available almost everywhere.

## It's right to give back if we can, but what isn't so widely talked about is how good it feels!

We all know it's right to give back if we can, but what isn't so widely talked about is how good it feels! As Ralph Waldo Emerson said, 'Serve and thou shalt be served.' Donate time or money to a charity not because you feel you ought to or because it makes you look good, but because you truly *want* to, and you really begin to see the abundance around you. You see that you can afford to fund a teacher in the developing world, or to help give a village clean water. That you have time to help others.

As we express mercy and compassion, so will we receive it. There is perfect balance in the law of karma. And sometimes all it takes is to share a smile and acknowledgement.

# TIP

## ALTERNATIVES TO SHOUTING

WHEN YOU FEEL yourself coming to the boil, stop. Wait one second. Think: am I going to be the same me, and get the same results? Or am I going to react differently, and see if something better happens? You already know that shouting and losing your temper doesn't work. So take a deep breath and try something different.

I've explored all the different ways. Like most of us, shouting was my first thing, but it didn't work. Next I tried to be calm, rational. But sometimes that didn't work either! In my family, what works best is if you're just silent. Nobody likes to be ignored. It doesn't take long before they say, 'Mummy, you're not talking! What have I done?'

Now the kids say to me, 'I hate that.' When that happens, I know I've really done it!

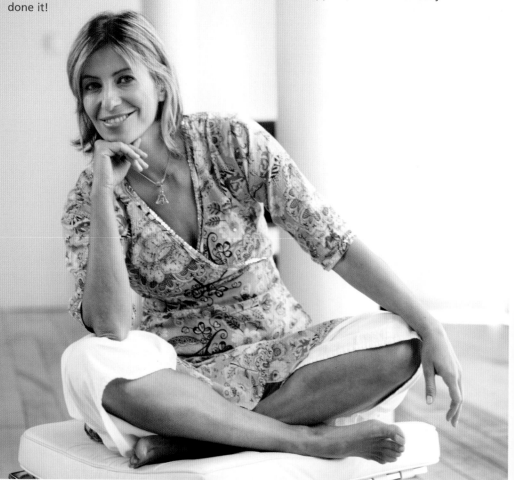

# RECIPE

## Visionizer

Mango is the king of fruits, rich in bioflavonoids, antioxidants, fibre and Vitamin C. This delicate shake activates the vibration of light, and when combined with the influence of blackberry, it will help you attain a sublime mind. Flaxseed oil (also known as linseed oil) is nature's richest source of omega-3 fatty acids, and, among its many health benefits, it can relieve arthritis symptoms, help prevent atherosclerosis (the accumulation of fatty deposits inside the blood vessels that many people experience as they get older) and improve mental function in older people. My kids love it, though they prefer it without the mint.

1 mango, stoned and chopped
175g (³/₄ cup) fresh or frozen blackberries
240ml (1 cup) filtered water
1 tablespoon chopped fresh mint leaves
1 tablespoon flaxseed oil

Place all the ingredients
in a blender and purée.

# EXERCISES

### Pregnancy Life Nerve Stretch

This exercise stretches the backs of your legs, your groin and your lower back, increasing circulation and flexibility. It also helps to keep your back strong throughout your pregnancy, relieves constipation and gas and relaxes your nerves. In yoga, we call the sciatic nerve along the back of the legs the life nerve, because of the effect stretching this area has on the entire nervous system. When you keep this area flexible, you release tensions in all areas of your body and mind, relaxing you deeply and improving your sleep. (And one thing you need during pregnancy is sleep – you'll get precious little of it afterwards!)

**A cautionary note: if you're already experiencing sciatica, which is inflammation of the sciatic nerve, do not do this stretching exercise until the pain is totally gone.**

Sit upright on the floor with your legs stretched out in front of you. Spread your legs two to three feet apart – or as far apart as you can. Make sure your spine is straight, then stretch your arms out in front of you, parallel to the floor. Inhale, and lean slightly back. Exhale and lean forward, stretching your arms and keeping them parallel to the floor. Create a rhythmic movement, mentally chanting, 'Sat' when you inhale, and 'Nam' (*naaam*) when you exhale. Continue for up to three minutes.

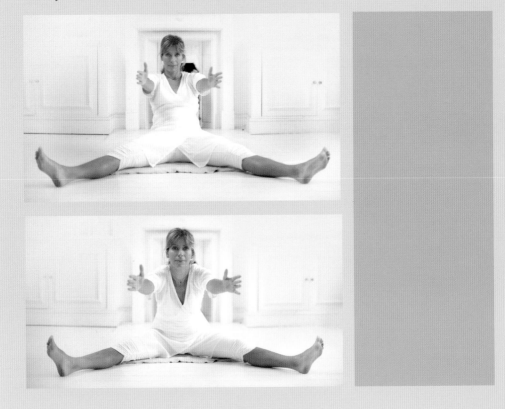

## Squatting (to prepare for birthing)

Squatting is a helpful exercise for pregnancy. Many women around the world find squatting the most comfortable position for giving birth, as well as for socializing and waiting for the bus! It is said that women who practise this posture their whole lives have a much easier time giving birth, as it increases flexibility and circulation of the pelvic area and strengthens and stretches your back and legs. You can squat to get down to floor level to pick something up, play with children, or when you need to bend over or lift something. Squatting also helps elimination, and it can help prevent constipation and haemorrhoids.

**Caution: Do not practise squatting if your doctor has indicated to you that your cervix is soft or open to full term.**

Begin with your back against a wall or with a sturdy chair in front of you for support. Squat down, and maintain the position for as long as is comfortable. Start with one minute a few times a day and build slowly. Take long, deep breaths, relaxing your body. Hold the chair for support. If you need to, place a folded towel or blanket under your heels for further support.

To come out of this squat, stand slowly so you don't get dizzy. You can also end by sitting fully on the floor. You can then relax, or stand up without the pressure on your knees.

# EXERCISES

## Pelvic Floor Exercises or Kegels

These simple exercises are helpful during pregnancy, and essential afterwards. All women should practise them regularly, and as we get older they can quickly help strengthen the muscles of the pelvic floor, preventing loss of urine during coughing or sneezing. Don't underestimate these common and simple exercises. Many women report increased strength after only a few weeks of practising them about fifty times a day.

Pelvic floor exercises can be done at any time. No one will know you're doing them. It's good to get into the habit of doing them in certain situations you encounter every day: waiting at the bus stop, for instance, or queuing in a shop.

To practise, sit comfortably and relax your breath. Tighten your bladder muscles as if you were stopping the flow of your urine, hold for a moment, then let go gradually. Think of this movement like an elevator, drawing the muscle up to the top floor, holding for a maximum of ten seconds, then slowly releasing, letting the elevator back down to the ground floor. Do these exercises as often as you wish. Practise after you have emptied your bladder.

# EXERCISES

## Hip Rotation

This stretches and loosens the hips to make birth easier, and also releases tension in the lower back, which is under so much pressure while you're pregnant – especially in the last trimester.

Crouching on your hands and knees, start to rotate your hips in circles. Continue in one direction for one to three minutes. Then pause, reverse the direction, and continue for another one to three minutes. Afterwards, relax into Child's Pose (see page 178).

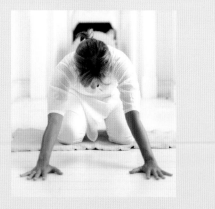

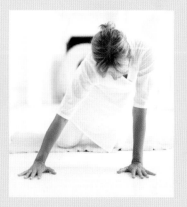

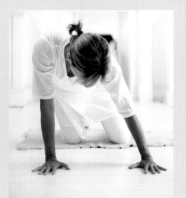

# EXERCISES

## Child's Pose

This is very similar to the position we take as babies in the womb, hence the name. It stimulates the pituitary gland, and helps you relax completely.

Start by sitting on your heels and spreading your knees, leaving room for your belly. Lean forward and rest your head on the floor. If it doesn't reach comfortably, rest it on a book. The important thing is that you let its weight rest on the floor or support, rather than holding it with your neck. Relax your arms by your side, near your feet, with your palms facing upward. Relax your breath and concentrate on your brow point, just between your eyes. If you are experiencing low or high blood pressure or you get dizzy, place a mat under your head, so that it does not go lower than your heart, or rest your head in your hands. Remain there for three to five minutes. Come out of this position slowly and relax for a few moments afterwards.

## Meditation to relax your baby

This meditation is a beautiful way to relax together. It's like having a spiritual conversation with your baby.

Sit in a comfortable meditation position. Hold your hands so that the thumb of your right hand rests in the palm of your left. Cross the thumb of your left hand over your right thumb. Relax your elbows by your side and raise both hands in front of your chest. Keep your eyes closed. Inhale a long, deep breath. On the exhalation, chant a long 'Saaaaat' (pronounced *su-au-u-ht*, as in 'but'). At the very end, when your breath is almost all out, chant a short 'Nam', just to let out the last bit of breath. Try to pronounce the 'Sat' thirty-five times longer than the 'Nam'. So *saaaaaaaaaaaaaaaaaaaaaaaaaat nam*. Inhale deeply and repeat the chant, allowing the breath to release slowly. Experience the sound. Don't struggle; let the sound be like a 'call'. Continue for three to thirty-one minutes. To end, inhale, suspend the breath briefly, then exhale and relax. In a short time, you can be breathing four to six breaths per minute, instead of the normal twelve to fifteen.

The long exhalation as you chant enables your breathing to slow down. Your body and mind receive a message of calm from your slowing breath rate, allowing you and your baby to relax. You will both fall in love with your voice, and the sound of your call! This is not just a meditation for new mothers, however. Try it any time, to help you find your balance and neutralize tension. It can help you bring your dreams and desires to fruition: visualize whatever it is you want during the meditation.

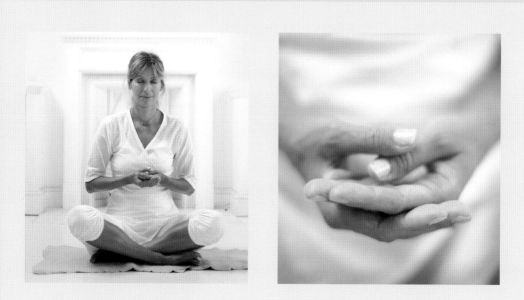

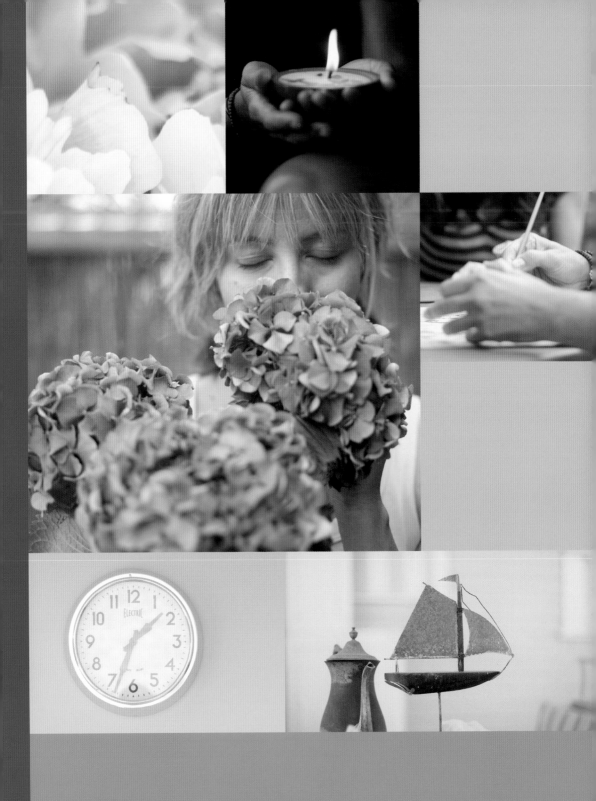

# Finding Joy

# CROWN CHAKRA

LOCATED AT THE CROWN OF THE HEAD, the seventh chakra is generally considered to be the centre of pure consciousness. It is linked to the pituitary gland, which secretes hormones that communicate with the rest of the endocrine system and also connects to the central nervous system via the hypothalamus. The thalamus is thought to have a key role in the physical basis of consciousness. This energy centre is associated with inner wisdom, our connection to a higher power, to the Universe or to our better selves.

There is an eighth chakra, the aura, which is the electromagnetic field that surrounds us like a halo. It's important that this is clear, as it is our connection to the upper realms, and everything that happens in our life is through that aura. So if it is strong, you are strong too. You're healthy emotionally, mentally and physically. Your immune system works better. Close your eyes and imagine a shield around you, a white or blue light. Put yourself visually in that space.

| GOVERNS: | SHADOW EMOTIONS: | COLOUR: | SYMBOL: | ELEMENT: |
|---|---|---|---|---|
| Boundlessness, connection | Grief | Blue | A lotus with 1,000 petals | None |

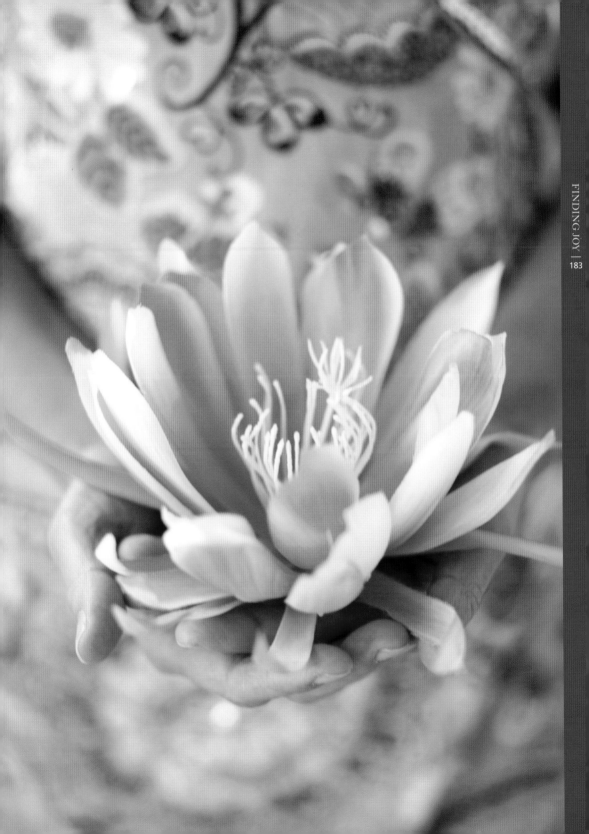

# Going deeper

'Go inside and listen to your inner voice. Every question has an answer. Your soul is full of wisdom and knows the way.'

YOGI BHAJAN (1929–2004)

I SOMETIMES LIKEN KUNDALINI to peeling an onion. Layer after layer comes away as we come closer to the core of our being, our authentic selves. It's your choice how far you go, and I'm not sure you're ever done – we keep learning right until the day we die. But as you peel those layers away, you'll notice subtle changes. What you eat, how you dress, what you say, how you react, what you want out of life, will shift – perhaps so slightly, at first, that you barely notice it.

My students share such experiences with me all the time. They find they are able to stop at just one glass of wine, and really savour and enjoy it, rather than finishing off the whole bottle in one sitting. They find they don't want that cigarette. Or that they no longer enjoy junk food, and the whole idea of sitting in the noisy, plastic environment of a fast food restaurant repels them. 'When I have cravings now,' says Jacqui, whose treat was once to eat two Big Macs, 'it tends to be for something like monkfish or seafood risotto. I'm just not eating processed foods any more, or having so many caffeine drinks.'

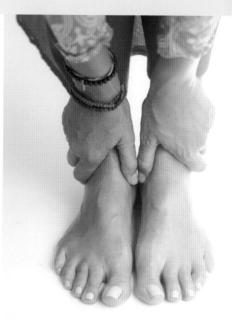

You might find you no longer enjoy gossip, or that you shy away from the water-cooler at work when you see people gathering for a good old moan. You might suddenly realize that friends who were always negative no longer seek you out, and that you've started to attract new friends who talk about their ideas and plans, who are keen to try new things, who make you feel alive. You might find, when you are snappy with to dance and start going out clubbing all night, revelling in their new-found energy and zest for life. There is no right and wrong way here. Yoga is a way of life, but that way is all about looking deep inside and finding the answers for yourself. There are no rules. It's up to you to decide.

What is certain, if you persevere with Kundalini, is that your skin will glow, aches and pains and other ailments will

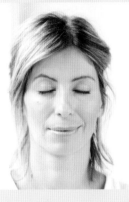

With Kundalini, your skin will glow, aches and pains and other ailments will cease to be a problem.

the kids one morning, that they look bemused, then ask, 'Mum, did you miss your yoga this week?' You will definitely start to slow down, to do things without stress or hurry – and oddly, you'll also find you achieve more.

I have one student who described herself as 'a disco girl – I would go out clubbing till 4 a.m. even in my forties'. After a few months of Kundalini, she said goodbye to late nights on sticky dance-floors, preferring to meet friends for lunch, go for walks and develop an interest in art instead. Others, however, remember how much they used to love cease to be a problem, you'll be calmer, healthier, happier. Our bodies have all the medicine they need – we just have to learn how to use it. Even people with serious health issues can gain a better quality of life by working with breath and meditation.

# You are the Guru – more thoughts about meditation

'What you think you become.' MAHATMA GANDHI (1869–1948)

We are starting to see huge shifts in our society. The economy is crashing, we're all suffering from information overload, life seems to go faster and faster. Yogi Bhajan predicted this would happen in the West in the run-up to the year 2012. Changes are coming faster and faster, and it's important to learn to be flexible, to be able to adapt.

Like computers, our brains can fry out. People suffer from depression and all kinds of mental conditions because we have too much information and don't know how to handle it – unless we use the tools that yoga gives us. We have to turn inward, into meditation. That five to ten minutes when you just sit in silence with nothing else going on in your head makes such a difference. Just download those thoughts from your brain for a few moments and allow it to rest. You're like a computer – if you don't clear it every so often, the hard disk gets full, it starts to slow down, and eventually it breaks down and doesn't work at all.

Allow that little voice deep within you to speak, and you'll have clear information, clear knowledge. You have the answers.

Many people would do anything not to be alone, not to sit for ten minutes. They get scared, lonely, they panic. People fill up their lives with all sorts of unnecessary things to avoid this stillness.

But it's important to acknowledge that we're born alone, and we die alone. Sitting by yourself is beautiful. Find the time and space, persevere, and you'll eventually get to an open, expansive place where you can see clearly your connection with the Universe, the life force, your god or goddess or your Higher Self. What we choose to call it is up to us. But it is a place of great peace, of real joy. This, above all, is what I wish for all of you as you read this book and use the tools within it.

If you feel ready to go deeper with your meditation practice, here are a few pointers. Much as I have learned from Yogi Bhajan and other wise thinkers, healers and life coaches, I have never felt it necessary to attach myself to any one person's ideology or to become a dogged follower of any supposed guru. There is an old proverb, 'Don't follow the guru – you are the guru.' I always tell this to my students. 'Take what is valuable, learn the tools, then share them again. Do not become attached to the person who gives you the knowledge, just the knowledge itself.'

We must never forget to trust the soul's instinct. The moment we seek our identity by becoming sheep in someone else's flock, we lose sight of the very essence we seek to illuminate – our human spirit. Shine for who you are.

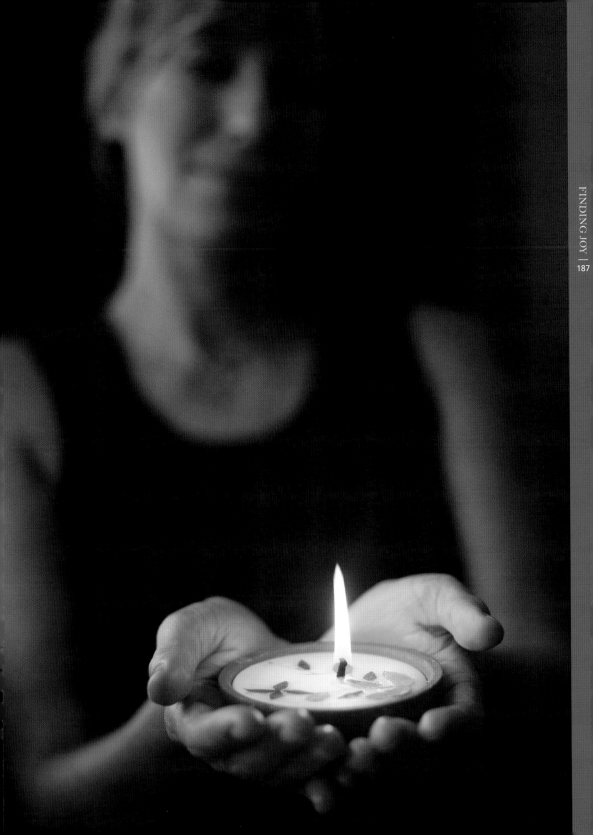

# Clothes

WEARING LIGHTER-COLOURED CLOTHES is believed to make your aura bigger and stronger. The white of the clothes we usually wear for Kundalini contains all the other colours, and symbolizes purity. It's up to you whether you choose to do this: you're after the teaching, not necessarily the tools that go with it.

However, if you wear the same clothes to your yoga classes or for your sessions at home it becomes like a uniform, full of the energy of what you do during that hour. That's why some people choose to wear robes for Kundalini – even as you're putting on the clothes, they remind you you're doing yoga and you feel different, calmer. It's the same when you put on sexy clothing – when you wear sexy clothing, you feel sexy, and you behave sexily.

I don't float around in white all the time. I've got lots of clothes I like, and I enjoy them! We have many characters inside us, many personalities, and they have to live together. My first Kundalini teacher, Shiv, on the other hand, put the robes on and never took them off. To him it's a reminder that this is the path he is living, and for him it's important to be reminded of that, all the time.

# Your meditation space

I WOULD LOVE TO HAVE A SPECIAL ROOM FOR MEDITATION, and if you have the space, go ahead and create one! For most of us, though, that's a luxury we can't afford. A corner of your bedroom will do, or any other room where you can find a quiet, clutter-free area. If your living space is tiny, just lay out your yoga mat, or use a meditation cushion. Going back to the same place every day helps your mind get to that space of deep meditation faster, because you know that when you sit here, this is what you do.

Ritual helps too. You might want to light a candle, or burn incense. Some people put a shawl round their shoulders to tell themselves they're now going into this mental space – useful if your corner is chilly!

You might want to make an altar on a shelf or low table. Collect a few pieces you love or find inspiring, and which give you peace. You might want to find a Buddha or some other religious icon. You could have a picture of your guru, your loved ones or yourself; a flower, some pebbles or shells from the beach, a piece of fruit or a glass of water – just something to say, 'I'm offering this time for myself. Just for this hour or this five or ten minutes, I'm doing this, for myself.'

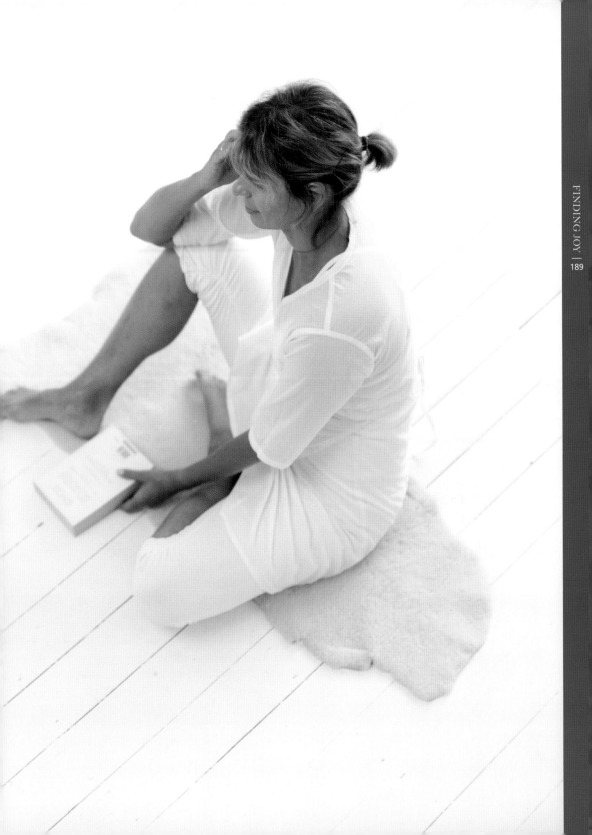

# The quest for joy

Right from when I was little I was always asking big questions that neither my parents nor teachers seemed interested in or had the time to answer. Where do we come from? Why are we here? Is there any greater purpose or meaning to life than school, work, marriage, babies followed by quiet old age? If this was all there was, I wasn't impressed.

'Happiness
is our
birthright.'
YOGI BHAJAN (1929–2004)

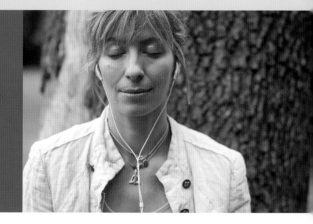

## Theres more to life than this...

Growing up in a boxy grey apartment block on the outskirts of a typically ugly Communist Bloc city like Skopje, everything seemed rather mundane. At night I would gaze up at the star-strewn sky and be certain I could feel the presence of a benevolent and loving energy looking down at me. Whenever I felt low, afraid or alone, I would share my thoughts aloud with the heavens, and always had the sense that I was listened to.

The quest that began with those conversations with the stars would stay with me into adulthood, when I dabbled with everything on the New Age market,

high on the hope that I would find the answers I sought. Convinced there had to be more to life than romance, partying and Jimmy Choo shoes, I embraced every Eastern philosophy and fitness fad going. I tried wearing a metal pyramid on my head to balance energies, I tried ancestor therapy, ozone therapy, goddess workshops, fasting, neuro-linguistic programming, urine therapy, dolphin-assisted therapy – and still most of these had little or no lasting effect on me. Nothing brought me closer to that simple sense of connectedness to a higher power that I had felt the potential for as a child.

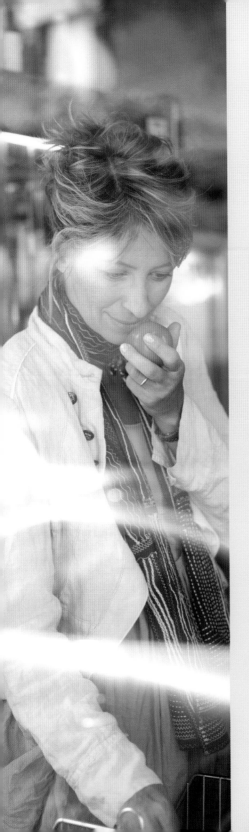

My open-mindedness was always counter-balanced by a typically Slavic no-nonsense mindset. My mother, of course, thought I was bonkers. When she came to visit me in London she became increasingly concerned. 'Have you joined a sect, dear?' she would ask me as I swirled sticks of sage around the apartment to ward off negative energy. 'It all seems like voodoo to me!'

I began practising yoga when I was twenty-five. My first studies were in Hatha yoga, then Ashtanga and Iyengar. I sweated it out in Bikram tents and danced my socks off to hip hop yoga. Although I learned much from each of these, they were paving stones on the path to the mother of all yoga, Kundalini.

I was always planning the next big thing in my life, but I was not mindful of the present, the Now. As John Lennon said, 'Life is what happens to you while you're busy making other plans.'

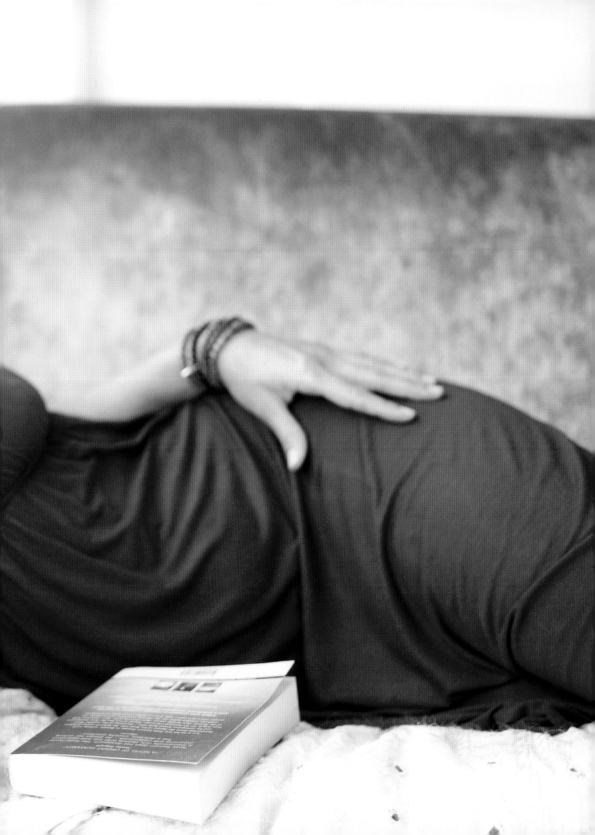

## Finding a Guru

A friend of my husband came to stay. Sean was a practising Buddhist, a recording engineer who had turned his back on the music industry. He came for a few weeks but stayed a year, helping out in the household, soon being nicknamed 'Monk Nanny' by our daughters. Sean sensed the unease that was eating away at me. 'Come and meet Shiv,' he said one day. 'He's not a therapist or guru – just someone incredibly tuned in who will listen and offer wisdom and advice.'

So I set off to meet Shiv in a dingy, one-bedroom flat up a rickety flight of stairs in a dilapidated house in the unfashionable part of deeply unfashionable East Finchley. He was an ex-junkie from Glasgow who wore the robes and turban of the Sikh religion. Skeleton-thin, with a straggly beard, he looked as if he had stepped out of a cave in the Himalayas. Glam guru he was not, but he read me like a book and his words touched me. Shiv's philosophy and life practice was Kundalini, and on his advice I began to attend classes.

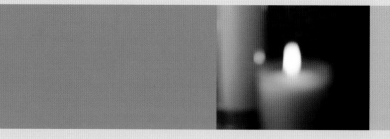

At first I thought it all a bit weird. The teacher spoke of a coiled serpent within us that we could learn to release and harness with incredible empowering effect. If my mother could see me now, I thought, chanting 'Wahe guru' with a room full of turbaned and white-robed strangers looking like extras from *A Handmaid's Tale* or *Rosemary's Baby*! I found the repetitive exercises and focus on breath and chanting strange; they made me dizzy and my limbs ached like crazy as I pushed through an eleven-minute exercise that pretty much consisted of flapping my arms frantically by my side like a bilious bird never destined to take flight.

But by the end of the first class, I'd got something. It was so direct, so powerful, that I felt it straight away. As a musician I loved the use of sound, the gongs and the prayer bowls and the mantra. So I carried on. I began to make space and time for myself, and realized for the first time how much I needed that.

Then, in the third class, it really kicked in. I felt my spirit and inner voice talking to me, much more clearly. We were chanting, we were sweating, and

I was so dizzy from the deep breathing I almost fainted. It feels like you're stoned or high, because of all the endorphins flooding your body. And then my mind shut up. For a few moments there, I didn't think. I was quiet. And I experienced the silence, and how it made me calm, relaxed. At that moment I realized, 'Wow! This is really giving me the whole picture. This gives me peace.'

It was an emotional moment, and I knew instantly that this was a path the Universe had chosen for me. Sean moved on, but I kept going to Kundalini classes. And in 2003, I started studying to become a Kundalini teacher. After two years of dragging myself out of bed at 4 a.m. at weekends to join the 5 a.m. meditation that started a day of Kundalini study, I received my diploma and my spiritual name, Harbajan, meaning 'Praise the name of the lord with sound'.

# At the heart of the teachings of Yogi Bhajan is the lesson of selflessness and the importance of giving back to the Universe all you receive from it.

## The pupil becomes the teacher

Twenty years ago, nothing could have been further from my mind than teaching! Even when I first decided to study Kundalini, I never thought of instructing others; I was fascinated with its blend of physical exercise, mystic teaching and science, and content to reap the benefits for myself. But at the heart of the teachings of Yogi Bhajan is the lesson of selflessness and the importance of giving back to the Universe all you receive from it. As he said when he came to California from India, 'I am not here to create students, but to create teachers.'

I feel very different from the career-centred person I was twenty years ago. You can live a life of seeing yourself in the mirror and never delving under the surface, but that's only the shell of what's inside. Whether you call it your soul, your spirit, God, your better self, your inner child, we all have a signature hidden within us. It's like a diamond buried deep – we have to get the mud off, clean it again and again until it's all glittering and shiny.

There are many ways through which we can get glimpses of our spirit souls: when we meet a life partner or soulmate and we sense a special connection; when a child is born and we feel in awe of the whole purpose of life; when a close friend or relative passes away and we feel their spirit still among us. Music, companionship, a beautiful sunset – they all give us a fleeting sense of this 'oceanic' feeling, but trying to keep this glimpse of the divine in our hearts is like trying to catch a butterfly without a net, or, in the words of Mother Superior in *The Sound of Music*, like trying to hold a moonbeam in your hands.

## ...and a whole new chapter.

The joy I have found in my yoga practice is something more permanent, something that stays with me, deep down. Ultimately, it's the joy of finding that connection with yourself. You don't need anybody when you're in that space. You feel content with your surroundings, and with everything around you. Finally you come to a point where nothing matters. You're not striving, you're not pushing, it's just OK. Inner joy is all about letting go and being content with who you are, and with everything around you.

We each have our own story, our own dreams, aspirations, flaws and failures, and we will each have our own personal experience of this quest for joy. But let's start by becoming conscious and respectful of our body as the vessel that carries us through life. Whether we are wheelchair-bound or athletic, we owe it to ourselves to remain in touch with the way our bodies work and to nourish and nurture them sensibly. If Botox or liposuction make you feel more self-confident, that's fine, but don't forget, it's a short-fix strategy. It's working for the ego, not the soul.

# Let life take its course. Let the sunshine in, let the soul come alive, let go – let God! This is joy.

Let us free ourselves of any stigma concerning our social standing or what possessions we own. To have been given the gift of life alone is extraordinary enough, and we should be grateful and humble. We should not be embarrassed to give thanks, regardless of our religious beliefs. The moment you remove yourself from the centre of the Universe (and it's hard, I know!) and acknowledge with thanks that you are blessed to be alive, is the moment you free yourself.

Let us learn to love our children, friends and family unconditionally, never judging, controlling or manipulating but with fair compassion and reason. Everyone we know is a bird in flight like ourselves, sometimes lost, often in need of protection but ultimately seeking their own truth.

Let us take responsibility for the world around us. We are all in this together, and the more we give service to others the richer we will feel for it. Being environmentally conscious in even the smallest way will make a difference. Be informed, not indifferent. And let us return favours whenever we can. From the simplest offer of taking on the school run for an overworked neighbour, to organizing a charity jumble sale/sky dive or volunteering to help out at the local old people's home.

Finally, let's try to relinquish control ourselves. Let's quieten our busy minds, through meditation, mantra, or simply a country walk, finding time to reflect and bask in the beauty of nature. Let life take its course. Let the sunshine in, let the soul come alive, let go – let God! This is joy.

### Divine Align
This light, sweet, refreshing drink will
connect you to your higher self.

¼ of a pineapple
175g (¾ cup) fresh or frozen blackberries
120ml (½ cup) fresh orange juice
1 teaspoon fresh ginger
2 teaspoons raw honey
dash of fresh lemon juice
pinch of cayenne pepper

Place all the ingredients in a blender and
purée. Serve with 'Wahe guru!'

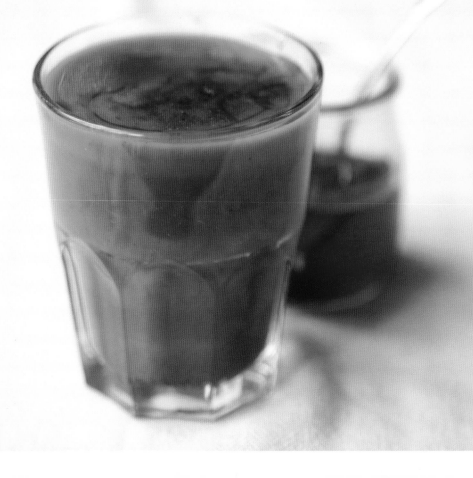

# EXERCISES

The following exercises will help you become more open to the benefits of meditation. Try different ones each time, or find the one that works best for you and stay with it.

## Moving Yoga Mudra

Sitting cross-legged in Easy Pose (see page 18), interlace the hands behind the base of the spine. Begin the Breath of Fire (see page 70) and bend forwards into Yoga Mudra by bringing the arms up and letting your head touch the ground. Then bring your head up. Continue to alternate positions and move at a steady pace in coordination with the breath for two minutes. When finished, release your hands and relax. If this is too challenging, place your hands on the floor in front of you instead, and bring your head slowly to the floor and back again, inhaling as you move up, exhaling as you move down. You can support your knees with cushions if that helps.

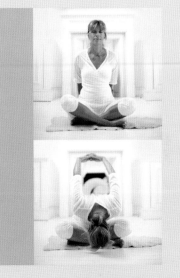

## Clear Your Thoughts

This is a nice easy warm-up for meditation.
Sitting cross-legged in Easy Pose (see page 18), interlace your fingers and put them behind your neck. Start a rapid movement with your arms by raising them up and down. Breathe powerfully through your nose for three minutes. This works on the main arteries to the brain, helping to bring you to deep meditation. Once your head is free from thoughts, you feel the space inside, which is bliss and joy. Relax your hands down and stay still for a while.

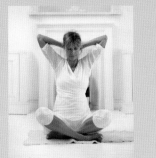

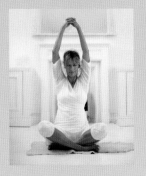

## Yogi Push-ups

Kneel on all fours, palms flat on the floor, fingers spread, toes tucked under and on the floor. Push up with your hips, keeping your legs and arms straight and the weight evenly distributed between your hands and feet.

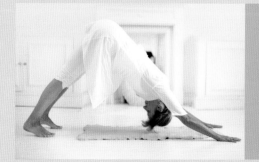

Your body should now be in an upside-down 'V' shape. This is Triangle Pose, or Downward Dog. Now, as you inhale, raise the left leg up with the knee straight. As you exhale, bend your arms, bringing your head to the ground. Inhale and come back to the original pose. Continue for one minute. Then switch legs for another minute.

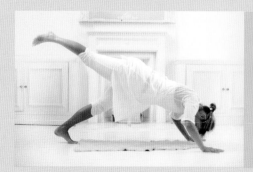

This is a very demanding pose but it will strengthen your crown chakra energy, opening it up to receive connection from your higher power. It's as if you are tuning your antennae into this higher frequency, setting you up for a really powerful and enlightening meditation.

Afterwards, sit in Easy Pose (see page 18) and relax your breathing.

## Lion's Paws

Sit down in Easy Pose, with your eyes closed. Open your mouth and breathe loudly through it, almost making an 'O' shape and sound. Curl your hands slightly so they look like a lion's paws, then sweep them up above your head. Inhale as they go up, exhale loudly when they go down. You're tracing an arc shape around your aura, making it stronger. Continue for one to three minutes.

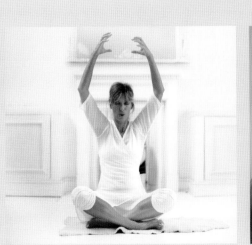

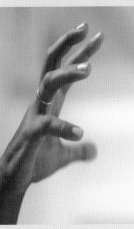

## Meditation for Guidance

With eyes closed, bring your elbows close to your ribcage and open your hands at a sixty-degree angle with palms up, as if ready to receive the guidance, offerings and protection of the Universe. Really feel the energy in your palms, almost like listening to the response from Infinity. Meditate for six minutes or more.

## Meditation for Abundance

Sit in Easy Pose (see page 18) with eyes closed, then open your eyes just a fraction and look at the tip of your nose. Put your hands in front of you, forming a cup. Keep your arms close to your ribcage. Meditate for as long as you want.

You will find that looking at the tip of the nose is not easy and will make you a bit dizzy. If that happens, just close your eyes and carry on with meditation. If you practise regularly, you won't feel the strain any more. It stimulates the optic nerve, the pineal gland and the frontal lobe of the brain – it literally controls the mind, making you calmer and helping to develop intuition. Soon the stillness and the silence within will become so loud that you won't hear anything or anyone else around you. You will begin to feel an immense sense of inner peace and joy. Imagine your hands open for blessings from Heaven: health, wealth, happiness and joy. Imagine all these and more pouring into your hands in abundance. Imagine anything you desire, and trust that you will receive.

You have opened the gateway and begun your journey of transformation, and you deserve the reward of ultimate joy!

# What next?

CLASSES

Details of Maya's workshops and retreats can be found on www.mayaspace.com.

The Kundalini Yoga Teachers Association lists classes all over the UK: www.kundaliniyoga.org.uk.

Maya's first teacher in London, Shiv Charan Singh: see www.karamkriya.com.

In London, Maya particularly recommends the classes at Alchemy Yoga and Meditation Studio, Chalk Farm Road, London, NW1 8AH (020 7267 6188).

For classes in Laughter Yoga (including telephone and Skype sessions!) go to www.laughteryoga.org.

STOCKISTS/TRAVEL

Devotion is a great general website for white yoga clothes and natural mats, mantra recordings, books and beautiful objects. All at www.devotion.co.uk.

Maya's own yoga mat is made from cork – a natural material with good antibacterial properties for hygiene. From www.stiilelibero.co.uk.

Maya likes the Italian-made LOVE aromatherapy shower gel collection, all-natural holistic products in four fragrances based on essential oils to suit your mood. You can order them online from www.officinadetornabuoni.eu.

Maya loves the COMO Shambhala retreats, but if you're unable to get out to Bali or Bhutan, they also sell spa products and a great range of white yoga clothing via their website, www.comoshambhala.como.bz.

Maya also warmly recommends the Carlisle Bay Hotel in Antigua, where she holds regular yoga retreats. www.carlisle-bay.com.

DVDs
*Kundalini Yoga to Detox & De-Stress with Maya Fiennes* (Acacia).

*Kundalini Yoga with Maya Fiennes, A Journey Through the Chakras. Courage, Creativity & Willpower* (Body In Balance) – Three DVD box set dealing with the lower triangle, the first three chakras.

*Kundalini Yoga with Maya Fiennes, A Journey Through the Chakras. Love & Truth.* (Body In Balance) – Two DVD box set dealing with the heart and throat chakras.

*Kundalini Yoga with Maya Fiennes, A Journey Through the Chakras.* (Body In Balance) Final box set to be released in late 2009.

CDs
MayaSpace, *Mood Mantras.*
Maya Fiennes, *MayaSpace.*
Both Maya's mantra CDs are available via her website, www.mayaspace.com.

Fans of Maya's music might also enjoy the mantras and music of US singer and Kundalini practictioner Snatam Kaur, see www.snatamkaur.com.

FURTHER READING
Deepak Chopra, *Kama Sutra* (London, Virgin, 2006). Beautifully illustrated book with translated extracts from the classic Indian book about sex and sensuality, and Chopra's own Seven Spiritual Laws of Love.

Thich Nhât Hanh, *Peace Is Every Step* (London, Random House, 1991). Collection of short speeches and writings by the Vietnamese Buddhist monk and teacher, encouraging us to use mindfulness in everyday life, from eating cookies or oranges to driving and answering the telephone.

Joseph Michael Levry, *The Divine Doctor* (Rootlight, 1993, out of print in the UK, but can be ordered from the US via Amazon.com). Yoga positions to help all kinds of illness.

Jelalu'ddin Rumi, *The Illustrated Rumi* (San Francisco, HarperSanFrancisco, 2000). The words of this Sufi mystic and poet still inspire and ring true 700 years after they were written.

Eckhart Tolle, *The Power of Now* (London, Hodder & Stoughton, 1999). Popular guide to being present and living in the moment.

# Glossary

**Asana** Another name for the positions in yoga. Each asana helps you become more aware of your body, mind and environment.

**Aura** Your aura is your protection, your shield. It is the electromagnetic field that surrounds your body.

**Body Drops** Sit in Easy Pose (see below), or with your legs straight out in front of you. Make your hands into fists, then start lifting your buttocks by pushing your fists into the ground and dropping down on to your sitting bones. Inhale as you go up, and exhale as you come down.

**Breath of Fire** A rapid inhale and exhale through both nostrils, just like sniffing; it is the best detoxifying breath. Its name comes from the purifying heat generated in the nostrils by the fast movement of air in and out.

**Bridge Pose** A position where you sit with your legs stretched out in front of you and place your hands behind you firmly on the floor. Breathe in and lift the buttocks, supporting yourself with your hands, with the body parallel to the ground. Let your head fall back.

**Cannon Breath** Pucker your mouth into a firm O shape and breathe through the mouth loudly, keeping your inhale and exhale equal, as in the Breath of Fire (see above). The name Cannon Breath comes from the sound your breath should make.

**Chakras** Energy centres which absorb life force from the Universe and distribute it to the nervous system, endocrine glands and circulatory system.

**Child's Pose, or Baby's Pose** A relaxing pose, just like a baby in the womb. Sit on your heels and rest your forehead on the floor.

**Cobra Pose** Lie on your stomach and raise your upper body up with your hands, palms on the ground. Lift your chest with your head back.

**Corpse Pose** The ultimate deep relaxation. Lie on your back, arms by your sides, with palms up. Relax completely.

**Cat–Cow Pose** Kneel on all fours, your knees directly under your hips, your hands level with your shoulders, index finger pointing forwards. As you inhale, curve your spine down towards the floor, and put your head back, looking towards the sky. As you exhale, arch your spine upwards and let your head hang down in a relaxed way, looking towards your navel.

**Crow Pose** Squat, with your feet apart.

**Downward Dog, or Triangle Pose** Stand with feet hip-width apart. Bend forward and place your hands on the ground, pushing your hips upwards. Keep your fingers spread wide. Your body should be in the shape of a triangle or upside-down V.

**Easy Pose** Sit with your legs crossed and back straight.

**Frog Pose** Squat on your toes, heels raised off the ground and touching each other, legs splayed out to the side like a frog. With eyes closed, place your hands on the ground and focus your attention on the third eye (see below). Breathe in and straighten your legs, raising your buttocks, hands remaining on the ground. Your heels should remain off the ground. Breathe out, and return to the squat.

**Guru** The inner teacher who helps us make the transformation from darkness into light.

**Gyan Mudra** Hand position where the index finger is touching the thumb to receive Divine Wisdom.

**Karma** In Hinduism and Buddhism, the principle of present life depending on past deeds.

**Kriya** A sequence of postures, breath and sound.

**Mantra** The sound vibration and rhythmical repetition of sacred words of empowerment, which elevate your consciousness.

**Prana** Life force, the energy we breathe.

**Root Lock, or Mulbandh** Contract the navel point, sex organs and anus to uncoil the Kundalini energy at the base of the spine.

**Rock Pose** Sit on your heels with hands on your thighs.

**Sat Kriya** Sit on your heels, or cross-legged in Easy Pose (see above) or on a chair. Stretch your arms above your head, touching your ears, with hands clasped together and index fingers pointing up. Close your eyes and focus your attention on the third eye (see below). Chant 'Sat!' loudly and sharply while pulling your navel in with a rapid, jerking movement. Then chant a longer, softer 'Nam' (*naaaaaam*) as you release your navel. Repeat for as long as you can.

**Third eye** The invisible point midway between your eyebrows.

**Venus Lock** Interlace your fingers, with the left thumb on top for women and the opposite for men.

**Yantra** A visual representation of your life.

**Yoga Mudra** Sitting cross-legged in Easy Pose (see above), interlace the hands behind the base of the spine. Begin the Breath of Fire (see above) and bend forward, bringing the arms up and letting your head touch the ground.

# Thank you!

There are so many wonderful and inspiring people I have met in my life, both through yoga and music, who have either supported me in my endeavors or in some way influenced and shaped me. I would like to take this opportunity to thank them all for their abundant and magical contribution to my life, all of which has enriched this book.

Special thanks must go to Camilla Richards for having such patience, unswerving belief, dedication and for creating the opportunity for me to write this book. My publisher Toby Mundy for getting it from day one. My editors, Caroline Knight and Sarah Castleton, for sharing and augmenting the vision for this book and acting as brilliant midwives, making its delivery smooth and painless. Sheryl Garratt for her eleventh hour alchemy and editorial flavour. Chris Shamwana for his inspiring design. David Loftus for capturing the essence in his photographs.

My teachers, especially Shiv Charan Singh who passed on such powerful truths with such humility, my students for their support and feedback, in particular those whose stories have been included in the book. Also to Deepak Chopra for his wisdom, insight and for giving me the confidence to put my thoughts down on paper.

My daughters Cheyenne and Shanti for giving me their time when time was precious, and for understanding 'this too will pass'. Now we're free to play again! Finally, a special thanks to Magnus for being such an unconditional resource of support and understanding, my wellspring of ideas and inspiration.